GEN-Z
PHARMACIST

Dominate
Pharmacy School
& Script Your
Dream Career

Adam Martin, PharmD

"A great tool for pharmacy students to utilize as they journey through pharmacy school and into the career field. While there are plenty of mentors in the field of pharmacy, now pharmacy students nationwide can have access to wonderful advice from a great mentor who loves helping others—Dr. Martin!"

>**Lindsay A. Morris, PharmD**
>2018 Next-Generation Pharmacist Award Winner
>Behavioral Health Clinical Pharmacist
>Department of the Army, Landstuhl Regional Medical Center

"This is a great book! A must read for all pharmacy students and those planning to enter the healthcare field."

>**Scott R Drab, PharmD, CDE, BC-ADM**
>Associate Professor of Pharmacy & Therapeutics
>University of Pittsburgh School of Pharmacy

"Reading and applying the principles from Gen-Z Pharmacist by Dr. Adam Martin will help you develop an intentional plan for personal and professional growth. Adam's passion and gift for inspiring others to become the best version of themselves comes through loud and clear in this book. This is a resource I wish I would have had available to me as a pharmacy student!"

>**Tim Ulbrich, PharmD**
>Clinical Professor of Pharmacy at The Ohio State University College of Pharmacy
>Co-Founder and CEO of Your Financial Pharmacist
>Co-Author of *Seven Figure Pharmacist*

"Whether you're a student in pharmacy school or a seasoned pharmacist, this book brings value to everyone. Dr. Martin provides multiple career options to help you find your best path to personal fulfillment and happiness. The self-care strategies, expectations for the future of the profession, exploring your dream job description, and so much more can all be found here!"

>**Michael Corvino, PharmD, BCPS, CDE**
>Clinical Pharmacist, Fetter Health Care Network
>Diabetes Educator, Palmetto Pharmacist Network
>Adjunct Assistant Professor of Pharmacology, CSU Physician Assistant Program
>Creator & Podcast Host, *CorConsultR$_x$*

"Pharmacy is rapidly changing, causing increased competition, but also opportunity for new grads. Gen-Z Pharmacist is an awesome tool for anyone in the profession looking to strengthen the skills needed for a competitive edge. The advice and lessons learned will be able to serve you well for years to come in your pharmacy career. Adam is truly passionate about what he does and it's great to see his ability to package and deliver a quality resource for pharmacy students. This is going to help a lot of people!"

>**Richard Waithe, PharmD**
>President, VUCA Health
>Author of *First Time Pharmacist*
>Creator & Podcast Host, *R$_x$Radio*

"Adam's positivity and energy shines through in his writing. He provides actionable advice and practical tips for aligning your life with your goals. This is a fantastic read for students who are striving for a more fulfilling life and career!"

Blair Thielemier, PharmD
Founder of BT Pharmacy Consulting, LLC
Founder of the Elevate Pharmacy Virtual Summit
Author of *How to Build Your Pharmacy Consulting Business*

"Dr. Martin's book is extremely well done. The minute I started reading it I was immediately motivated and informed on how to maximize my overall success. There are numerous key takeaways and exercises within the book that you can start implementing into your daily routines to improve your life. I personally have already started using a few of his time management tips and find myself having extra hours in the day, as well as an increase in productivity at my pharmacy. I wish this book was written sooner! It not only teaches about how to succeed in the world of pharmacy, but just life in general! This is a must read for anyone in the field of pharmacy!"

Joshua Stoneking, PharmD
National Director, 503A Oncology, Avella Specialty Pharmacy

"Gen-Z Pharmacist gives pharmacy students the encouragement to live a healthier lifestyle by reinforcing that, as healthcare professionals from whom patients seek health advice, we should be leading by example. This book lays out practical reasons and simple steps for you to take towards better physical and mental health. Read this book if you're ready to shift your life and become more effective....NO MORE EXCUSES!"

Hillary Blackburn, PharmD
Founder, Pharmacy Advisory Group
Creator & Podcast Host, *Talk to Your Pharmacist*
Founder & CEO, Natural Products Resource Center

"While each day the pharmacy community keeps healthcare top of mind, our own self-care tends to take a backseat. In this comprehensive volume, Adam Martin shows how you can take a both/and approach to your own wellbeing, which will improve the patients' as well. The book is a ready preventative and antidote to burnout."

Tony Guerra, PharmD
Pharmacology and Chemistry Professor, Des Moines Area Community College
Author of *Memorizing Pharmacology: A Relaxed Approach*

Copyright © 2020 by Adam Martin, PharmD
All rights reserved.

No part of this publication may be reproduced, distributed, or transmitted in any form or by any means, including photocopying, recording, or other electronic or mechanical methods, without the prior written permission of the publisher, except in the case of brief quotations embodied in critical reviews and certain other noncommercial uses permitted by copyright law.

ISBN 978-1-7326357-3-9

THE FIT PHARMACIST

Contents

Foreword viii

In Memoriam x

Part I: Your R$_x$ to Dominate Pharmacy School 1

(S) Self Mastery 2

    1. Clarify Your Why 3
    2. Mold Your Mindset 9
    3. Self-Care = Healthcare 15
    4. Tame Time Management With Deep Work 27
    5. Ask for Help PRN 37
    6. The Value of an Outside Passion 43
    7. Building Your Personal Brand and Your Competitive Edge 49

(R) Relationship Building 60

    8. Master Your Emotional Intelligence 61
    9. Nurture Your Networking 73
    10. The Three Levels of Mentorship 87
    11. Leadership & Legacy 93
    12. Build Your Team as a Pharmacy Leader 97
    13. Dispense Your Full Potential as a Leader 103
    14. The Long Game 109

Part II: Script Your Career—Experts Speak **115**

    22 Formulas for a Fulfilling Career 117

    Specialty Pharmacy 119

    Community Pharmacy I 126

    Community Pharmacy II.. 130

    Residency... 135

    Business in Pharmacy 142

    Diabetes Care/Certified Diabetes Educator (CDE) 147

    Research I 152

    Research II 157

    PharmD to PhD Track.. 162

    Academia... 173

    Administration in Academia 178

    Administration in Community Pharmacy 183

    Managed Care 187

    Pharmacy Law 191

    Geriatric Pharmacy 194

    Geriatric Pharmacy as a Community Pharmacist................... 199

    Nuclear Pharmacy 203

    Infectious Disease... 208

    Medication Therapy Management 212

    State and National Organizations 219

    Creating Your Own Career as a Dream Business 225

    R_x Filled: MY Dream Pharmacy Career!.........................225

Acknowledgments... **232**

Resources **234**

Chapter References **235**

About the Author... **241**

"**I promise** to devote myself to a lifetime of service to others through the profession of pharmacy. In fulfilling this vow:

- I will consider the welfare of humanity and relief of suffering my primary concerns.

- I will apply my knowledge, experience, and skills to the best of my ability to assure optimal outcomes for my patients.

- I will respect and protect all personal and health information entrusted to me.

- I will accept the lifelong obligation to improve my professional knowledge and competence.

- I will hold myself and my colleagues to the highest principles of our profession's moral, ethical, and legal conduct.

- I will embrace and advocate changes that improve patient care.

- I will utilize my knowledge, skills, experiences, and values to prepare the next generation of pharmacists.

I take these vows voluntarily with the full realization of the responsibility with which I am entrusted by the public."

—Oath of a Pharmacist

Foreword

I wanted to be a pharmacist so badly! I felt that I was destined to do it, but there was just one problem: I was rejected from pharmacy school.

A year later I reapplied, only to end up on the waitlist. I was the last person to be accepted into my pharmacy school class of 2012. Fun fact: no one I graduated with knew this before now.

Despite these setbacks, I went on to become the president of my class, served in every leadership position in the Student National Pharmaceutical Association (SNPhA), was the publicity chair for Phi Delta Chi, was inducted into the Phi Lambda Sigma leadership society, and was awarded a $10,000 scholarship by the dean for being who she deemed "the most likely to innovate the profession of pharmacy." When you face adversity, KEEP GOING, DO NOT QUIT, and above all else, NEVER SETTLE for anything less than your best.

If I can do this, I know that *you* can. I want you to know that if you feel in your heart this is what you were meant to do, you have everything to be successful. After that, it is not about what resources you have, but about *how resourceful you can become*. And that is what we'll be covering in this book: how to make the most out of your time in pharmacy school, maximize your networking skills, learn from the absolute best in the profession to set up your accelerated career path, and not just survive school, or thrive, but to *dominate* your niche by living up to your full potential.

I was awarded a great privilege when I was accepted into pharmacy school. Once I earned admittance, I made the decision to make the most out of every single day by accomplishing just two things: to learn as much as possible both in and out of the classroom, and to have a positive impact on every single person with whom I interacted. With that mindset, work ethic, and commitment, pharmacy school became the most valuable four years of my life. I want you to have that same level of experience, if not more.

I am now a licensed and practicing pharmacist. Looking back on my time as a pharmacy student, I've realized that I became a part of a school that consistently gave so much value and support to its students that I want to give back, but not just a one-time gift. Volunteering and monetary gifts are great, and both are highly recommended and welcomed with open arms and appreciation, but I want to go even deeper. I want to leave an impact on current and future students at the University of Pittsburgh School of Pharmacy in a way that reflects how much I appreciate my time in pharmacy school. I want to serve those who now sit in a seat in which I worked so hard to sit. That's why I wrote this book: to help empower every pharmacy student. I include the greatest minds in our profession, to whom the second half of this book is dedicated. They have shared their wealth of knowledge and insight into how you can master your niche and endlessly fuel your passion in this profession to better serve your patients, community, world, and self. I want you to dispense your full potential.

In Memoriam

You have cancer. It is spreading and you have less than six months to live.

This was what my mother was told, which I was not made aware of until after her passing. While I think of her every day, and miss her dearly, her battle against cancer was what led me to the profession of pharmacy. I witnessed a genuine level of care and humanity toward her from a pharmacist, who was a total stranger to us. That pharmacist went above and beyond to ensure that all of her questions were answered and extended a level of service beyond what was expected just because it was the right thing to do as an advocate for her health. All of this, from a total stranger with no prior connection or ulterior motive. This stranger was who I wanted to become. So I began my journey into the profession of pharmacy. While my mother ended up fighting for more than five years, despite her less than six-month diagnosis, she passed away before I was finally accepted into pharmacy school. She taught me about the power of attitude, about why serving others should come first above all else, and how the level of impact you provide far outweighs any monetary compensation. Positively changing someone's life is simply *priceless*.

Please know that while you may have paid for this text, a substantial amount of the proceeds from this book go directly to an endowment fund at the University of Pittsburgh School of Pharmacy toward a scholarship for a passionate pharmacy student looking to innovate the way we practice pharmacy. This is one way I am giving back to the institution and profession that has given me so much. I hope one day to make a dent in the feeling of indebtedness to my alma mater for taking a chance on this student of life.

You may not have been there when I was accepted, but I fully dedicate this book and all of the passion herein to you, Mom. You are the reason I am who I am, and why I always strive to be a better person for those in my life. We were two peas in a pod, and the seeds of your love continue to bear fruit for others.

To you, Mom, and all the future pharmacists who will benefit from the following text as a result of your love and dedication to your son.

With eternal love,
Adam

PART I

Your R$_x$ to Dominate Pharmacy School

(S) SELF MASTERY

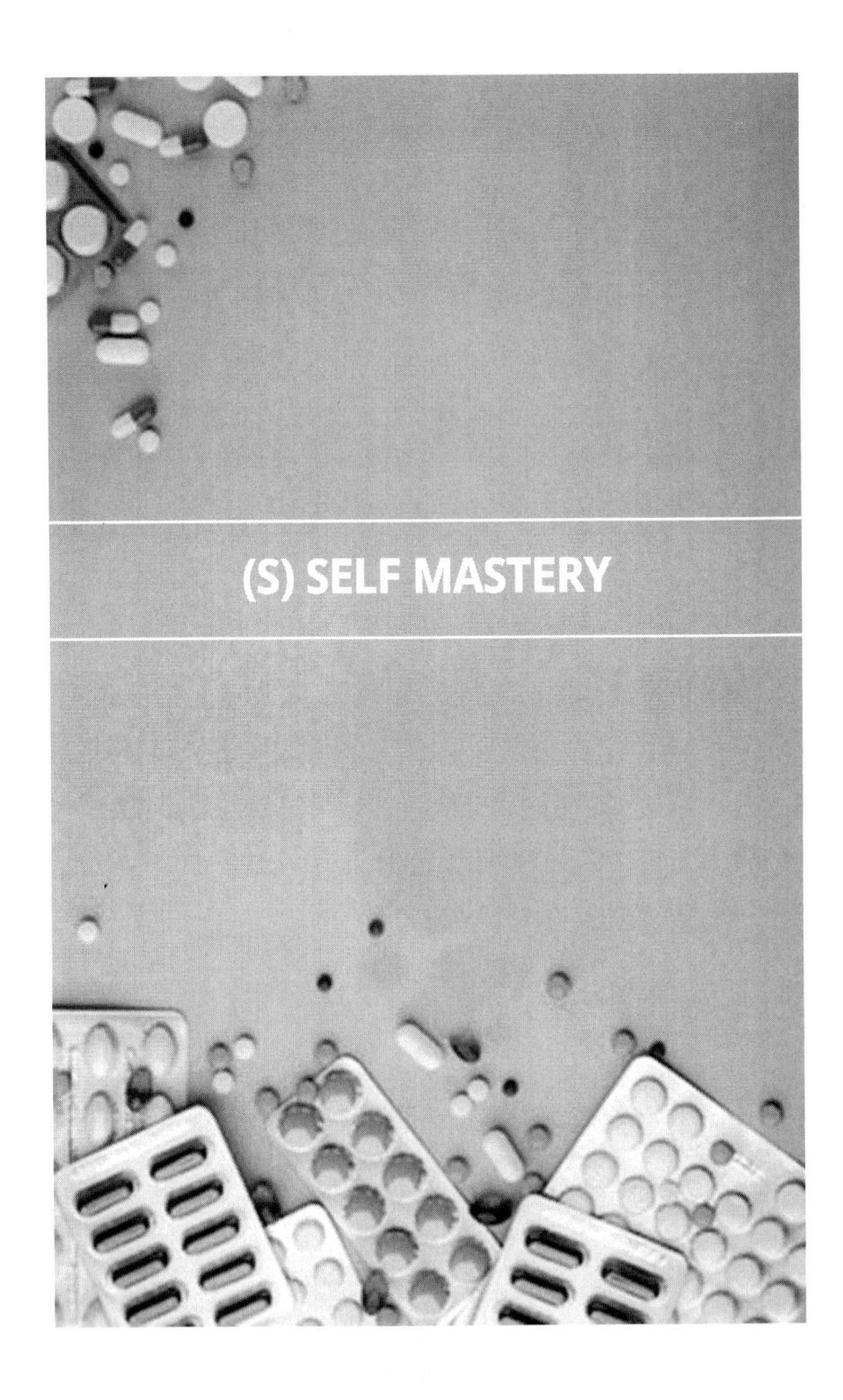

Chapter 1

CLARIFY YOUR WHY

"He who has a why to live can bear almost any how."

—Friedrich Nietzsche

I'M GOING TO take a stab here and guess that you didn't just pick pharmacy school with a dart board of specializations in high school. You didn't randomly glide through the pre-requisite classes, the PCAT exam, and the entire PharmCAS process with the countless hours, monetary cost, and sacrifice to get to the point where you clicked the submit button on your pharmacy school application. You had a *why*. You had a *reason* that you picked the pharmacy profession, and I'm going to go out on a limb here and guess that your reason is part of *your story*!

Here is a truth: we all have a story. You, me, your professor, your idol, and the homeless man you pass every morning on your commute. Here is another truth: *the majority of people keep that a secret*. Whether it's shame, not feeling good enough to share it, fear of rejection, or being ostracized for being real, vulnerability is a huge gamble. Many let fear of failure grow so strong in their minds that it silences their greatest asset! The real kicker is that, in keeping quiet, you are suppressing something that is actually an inspiring story that would resonate with many and bring you respect, rapport, and self-empowerment. Sadly, the fear of rejection that can be crafted by our inner Debbie Downer can sometimes feel so real that our story is never told. Our why is often kept in the shadows, locked away in a place that cannot fuel us to our full potential or help others find *their* inner voice.

Here is my challenge to you, and your first step in unleashing your inner power, your voice, your purpose—your why: *write your story down!* I can fully respect that you may be dealing with a searing level of pain, hurt, or impact that your story has had on your life. It may be so fresh that it brings you to tears, or even causes you to feel like an outcast. You may fear that by sharing it others will judge you or treat you differently. If that is the case, I encourage you to keep working through it. You can overcome any situation and cease to be a victim of circumstance. You can keep your written story to yourself, for your eyes only, if you wish–the key is to start with this one action: writing it down. *The pen is mightier than the sword*, as they say.

> But, Adam, if everyone has such a great story, why do so few people share it?

The number one reason people choose to not share their story with others, regardless of the specifics, is *fear*. I listed some versions of how fear is felt or displayed above, but it all boils down to that one thing: fear. So, how do we overcome it?

I am a pharmacist, after all, so knowing the best R_x of choice for a condition, disease, or infection is part of my job. Call it knowing the antidote for the condition, if you will. If you can master your mindset and free yourself from fear, imagine the endless possibilities that lie ahead in your future!

We've all heard the advice *live each day like it was your last*, but why is that so important? It's because, if you know that today is your last day to live, you have no fear. You have no mental blocks holding you back, no what-ifs jumping into your mind to stop you from trying this or trying that. *Nothing is standing in your way!*

Even if you fail big, it won't matter because this is literally your last day! You may not have thought about this cliché that deeply, but I want to show you how you can apply that logic and mindset to overcome your fear of sharing your story and ultimately your why. This is related to the part of my job as a pharmacist regarding knowing the best antidote—the solution—for a condition, this one being fear. I have learned one simple truth on my own personal journey: *the antidote to fear is ACTION.*

This is so true, my friends, I cannot stress it enough. No, it won't be comfortable, or even pleasant. Actually, it will more than likely even be *painful*! But imagine the freedom you'll feel if you are no longer a slave to fear.

ACTION is the antidote to fear.

I'm not asking you to step on a stage, to give a sermon or testimonial, or to yell your story from your window. Let's keep it just to you, for your eyes only. This is your story, and it is personal. It is impactful. It is unique because it is about *you*! I simply invite you to write down your story on these next few pages, just a paragraph or a couple sentences.

The challenge, if you choose to accept it, is to *ACT* by taking *ACTION*. I've left these next few pages blank and dedicate them to you and your why. I want to paint the picture of purpose and let you know that you matter! You are worthy of owning your story and becoming the author of your own life. You have the pen, the paper, and, being a pharmacy student, the purpose of starting on your journey toward impacting the lives of potentially millions of patients who you have the opportunity to serve. Owning your why and unleashing the power of greatness within you. It all starts with your *why* and the *actions* you choose to take by either leaving that a secret or tapping into your inner greatness and sharing it with the world. You have the blank pages. You have the pen. You have your story. Let's get this party started!

MY WHY

By _____

Date _____

I chose to study pharmacy because:

_____

_____

_____

_____

_____

_____

_____

_____

_____

_____

_____

_____

_____

_____

_____

_____

_____

Congratulations! You have just taken your first step in coming into your own power and fully developing into the very best future pharmacist you can be by owning your truth. This is for you! Maintaining your why at the forefront of your day as a pharmacy student will keep you focused throughout your journey. Developing a strong mindset along that journey when the storms of life strike will keep you on your path toward greatness. The *how* for molding that mindset is what we will explore next.

Chapter 2

MOLD YOUR MINDSET

"As you think, so shall you become."

—Bruce Lee

STAYING FOCUSED on what is most important to you will empower you. How? Shifting your focus and energy to simply control the controllables will gift you with a sigh of relief as you spend less of your time worrying about the rest—that which you can*not* control.

When you release these things, you also release all of the tension, anxiety, worry, and unnecessary energy spent on them so that you can instead invest in things that will serve you.

When you do this, you are practicing an act of self-care, which is all too often ignored by all of healthcare. You cannot pour from an empty cup. So let's dive into this foundational practice of greatness that will unveil the secret formula to becoming the best healthcare practitioner you can become!

Mindfulness is a huge buzzword right now, but what is it exactly? How do we use it? Does practicing it automatically make me a hipster?

Simply put, mindfulness is the act of paying attention. As healthcare professionals, we cannot perform well without doing a multitude of things at the same time: counseling patients, answering the phones, consulting with our co-workers, managing our teams, documenting our interactions—the list never ends! What about outside of work? Is living that way all the time, in every situation, really healthy for our long-term health? No!

The act of mindfulness is making an effort to focus on only one thing at a time. You read me right: *monotasking*. At face value it is simple, but data points to the real-life benefits that this practice can produce. Even when you're not actively practicing mindfulness, if you commit to making this a daily habit, you will see benefits. Don't miss the power in the simplicity of that statement!

> But, Adam, I have all of these things to do as a pharmacy student, let alone trying to live life, and you're telling me that doing less will help me to do more? I'm sorry, but I need more than your word that this will actually work!

Proof? The American Psychological Association cites mindfulness as "a hopeful strategy for alleviating depression, anxiety, and pain." It doesn't stop there. This mental practice can moderate the brain's amygdala, that classic fight-or-flight response center, based on research conducted at the University of Pittsburgh (hail to Pitt!) and Carnegie Mellon University. In essence, practicing mindfulness will reduce excessive stress over not-so-life-threatening events, like choosing where to eat dinner (Chipotle is the clear answer anyway).

Methods to Mindfulness

- **Meditation**

    You don't have to spend hours a day to experience the benefits of this activity—you can start with just ten minutes a day! Get a feel for the exercise and build on it from there. Research from a 2014 study at Carnegie Mellon found "three twenty-five-minute meditation sessions per week could alleviate stress."

    New to the art of meditation? There are plenty of free mobile-friendly apps that can guide you through the process! My top four at the time of this writing are Headspace, Calm, Whil, and Insight (if you're more advanced). Headspace is the best place to start, in my experience.

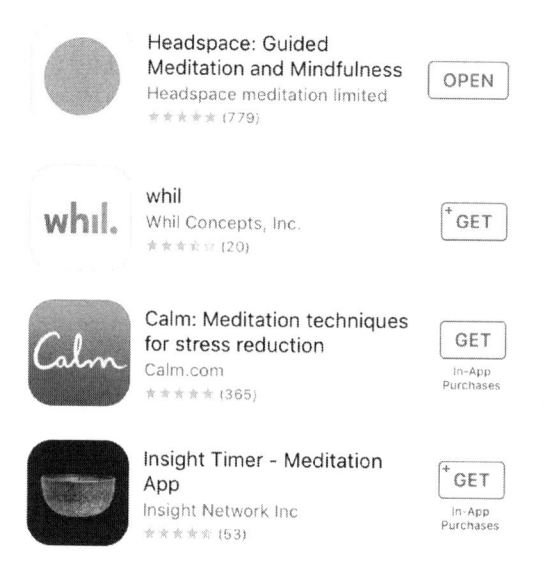

	Headspace: Guided Meditation and Mindfulness Headspace meditation limited ★★★★★ (779)	OPEN
whil.	whil Whil Concepts, Inc. ★★★★☆ (20)	+GET
	Calm: Meditation techniques for stress reduction Calm.com ★★★★★ (365)	GET In-App Purchases
	Insight Timer - Meditation App Insight Network Inc ★★★★☆ (53)	+GET In-App Purchases

- **Deep rhythmic breathing**

This might seem super simple, but do not underestimate this amazing tool. You can even use it during the crazy hustle and bustle at ClubPharmacy if you feel your stress levels climbing too high. *Trust me, I'm speaking from experience!*

There are many methods out there, but the basic concept is this:

1. Inhale deeply and slowly through your nose with the purpose of completely filling your lungs with air.

2. Pause for a brief moment, holding your breath.

3. Exhale deeply and slowly through your mouth with the purpose of emptying all the air from your lungs.

If you're able to (i.e., not in the midst of a stressful scenario), count your breaths to give focus to what you are doing, making this your only objective (monotasking!).

Count one with the inhale, two with the exhale, three with the inhale—up to a count of ten—then repeat PRN.

A helpful video that will guide you through this process in the resources section of my website, thefitpharmacist.com/resources.

- **Gratitude**

Focusing on what you are thankful for is the easiest, fastest, and cheapest way to kick start your positivity! Start your day off by physically writing down the things that you are thankful for in your life.

BONUS: Do you have a loved one? Do this with them—they will benefit, and it will likely highlight blessings you may have overlooked.

- **Exercise**

You don't have to be a bodybuilder to receive benefits from exercise. You can start with ten-minute exercise intervals if you're super crunched for time. Keep it going and build from there. Research from the University of California, San Francisco has shown that "forty-two minutes of vigorous activity over a three-day period can reduce stress on your telomeres." That's right, it can prevent aging at the cellular level!

- **Sleep!**

Struggling to hit the hay? The root cause may be your sleep hygiene—yes, there is such a thing! Ambien® isn't always the answer (that's coming from a pharmacist). There is a host of tips and tricks for this all-too-common issue, also found in the resources section of my website.

EXERCISE

Using the list of examples we just described, write down all of the things that you worry about on a daily basis. **Do not skip this step**! By physically writing them down, you are giving both voice and awareness to them so that you can then take action on them rather than allowing your thoughts to take control of you.

Thoughts and worries that frequently occupy my mind:

(example: passing my exam, wanting people in my class to like me, and my physical health and fitness)

_____

_____

_____

_____

_____

_____

_____

_____

_____

_____

_____

_____

_____

Now, looking at the list you made on the previous page, circle the specific thoughts that you can directly control and impact from your own actions and draw an "X" across those that you cannot control. Using the above example, you would circle *my physical health and fitness* as you can take actions to improve those, but you would draw a big "X" across *wanting people in my class to like me*, because you cannot control what other people think of you. Don't waste your time worrying about things you can't control; spend that energy on your health, FitPharmFam!

Hopefully you can now see the importance of mindfulness in your mental mojo and have some ideas on how you can improve it. Molding your mindset will allow you to maintain your focus and energy on the things that best serve you! This is the epitome of practicing self-care, which leads us right into our next chapter...

Chapter 3

....

SELF-CARE = HEALTHCARE

"If you're not growing, you're dying."

—William S. Burroughs

AS A PHARMACY STUDENT reading this book, I hope that you are hungry for success and that you want to become the very best version of yourself. Trying to do this on top of everything else in pharmacy school can leave you feeling like there aren't enough hours in the day! There are so many things to prioritize that *everything* may seem to be a priority and must be done now! Something has to give with this mentality, and if your own self-care is not a clear priority, this is often the first thing to go on the I'll-do-it-later list. Let me paint a picture of that risk:

Have you ever been thirsty? It's a silly question. We have all been thirsty at some point in our lives. The human body is an amazing system—it can survive twenty-one days without food, but only three days without water. So let's say you're studying for an exam at your library and you're super focused—I'm talking *in the zone!* You start to feel a little bit thirsty, but you have so many more chapters to review, you just keep trudging on. The feeling of thirst continues to swell (meta pun) until you become really thirsty. Now you also feel hungry, which starts to draw your focus away from studying. Right at the moment when you decide it's time to address these feelings, your good friend comes to sit next to you. After saying hi, she tells you that she's really thirsty and is wondering if you have a bottle of water to share. You're thirsty too, but you have nothing to offer.

In her time of need, she asked you for help, and you have nothing to offer her because you yourself are thirsty. Your cup is empty!

This may be a trite example, but I hope the message is clear. We all strive to give and serve others, but if we don't take care of ourselves first, we'll have nothing left to give!

The Most Important Formula
You Will Ever Learn as a Pharmacist:

Self-Care = Healthcare

As one of the most accessible health care providers, our patients come to us seeking advice not only for prescription medication and OTC questions, but also on the big question like *how do I get healthy?*

When I was in pharmacy school, I noticed something profound in all of my classes. Nutrition is the cornerstone of therapy for literally every single disease state we treat as healthcare professionals. However, even with all of the medications and invaluable information we learn and focus on in the limited time frame we have in school, we are not given much training on the science behind it. Patients will come to you frequently asking questions related to nutrition, so what are you going to say? Are you using those tips yourself? Are you leading them to better health by example, inspiring their journey?

In healthcare, we strive every day to improve the lives of those we serve. Sometimes we can care so deeply and give so much, that *we do so at the sacrifice of our own health*. It often starts small—skipping a meal or forgoing that one workout. For a one-time sacrifice, this doesn't seem like a big deal. However, if you continue to make these cuts day after day, over time this practice will become a habit that results in an unhealthy lifestyle. We can literally fall into the trap of sacrificing our own health because we think it's a dichotomy: to serve our patients best, we have to forgo our own health practices.

> But, Adam, I want to give one hundred percent and every moment of my time for the care of others.
>
> My full and undivided attention is a must.
>
> If I'm fooling around with meal prepping, working out, and sneaking in a quick meal, that's not serving my patients fully.
>
> Cooking and working out? I can't be that selfish! Working on fumes is expected—it's just part of the job.

I heard these beliefs throughout pharmacy school, both from students and from extremely passionate healthcare providers. They lived and practiced it, feeling that by sacrificing their own wellbeing, they were giving all of their passion and commitment to their patients. *They were the ultimate healthcare provider.* Want to know what else I noticed about these same individuals?

They often smoked to curb the stress.

They would commonly binge eat after work.

Both their professional and personal lives were ruled by anxiety and overwhelm.

The longer they had practiced these self-sacrificing beliefs, the more weight they would visibly gain, the darker the circles under their eyes grew, and the more exhausted and zombie-like they seemed in their day-to-day movements.

The most striking thing I noticed about those who had adopted this seemingly unselfish mentality was that *they felt less and less fulfilled as time went on.*

If you want to make this a lifelong career and not just a temporary job that you are forced to leave due to burnout, *I implore you* to shift from a self-sacrifice to a self-care mentality. You cannot pour from an empty cup. Take care of yourself first so that you can empower yourself to help others to your full potential!

As I graduated and became a full-time pharmacist living that high-workload lifestyle, I started to see this more and more. I thought to myself, *there's got to be a better way!* How can we, as healthcare providers, not live up to the standard that we are preaching to our patients?

This question repeated in my head year after year. I finally took action, not just for myself, but for my profession, which has given me so much and has enabled me to impact the lives of those I am blessed to both serve as patients and work with as colleagues. It led me to create The Fit Pharmacist movement: my own business, brand, and representation of myself as a pharmacist in our profession and healthcare community. This idea first sparked into my mind back when I was a P2 seeking a mentor for this ideology of combining fitness and pharmacy. I met with the pharmacy school dean, Dr. Patricia Kroboth, who said the following words to me that prompted my journey into innovation:

"Well, that doesn't yet exist—but you can create it."

I wanted to be an example for patients, friends, and family—someone who could empower and support them through their own journey into living their best lives. I didn't want this to stop at my role as a pharmacist. I wanted to live a healthy lifestyle that is practical, realistic, and simple—so simple that *any* healthcare professional could do it without having to follow a restrictive meal plan or rely on expensive supplements.

I've tried many strategies over the years, trying to gain muscle and trying to lose fat. In the end, I found it took a lot of time to even come close to reaching either. It can be extremely confusing to try to figure it out on your own. One health book, fad diet, or a guru says to eat fat, the other says only carbs, while the media says avoid both and the internet is telling you to eat only protein.

Amidst that frustration was where I found a concept known as flexible dieting, perfected and popularized by my good friend Joe Klemczewski, PhD, founder of The Diet Doc, LLC. Joe has helped the nutrition industry abandon the belief that, in order to get extreme results, I have to make extreme sacrifices!

Yes, you *can* have your cake and eat it too, without feeling guilty, restricted, or reliant on a supplement, product, or ___ [insert MLM company name]. This is honestly the answer that I feel everyone should understand. The answer isn't to rely on overpriced shakes, magical potions, or wonder gadgets that will solve all of your problems yesterday if you sign up today. *No product will replace the most effective tool you have: you!*

There's so much noise out there on nutrition—no wonder we're all confused—but it doesn't have to be so complicated. Nutrition can be super simple, it can be enjoyable, and it can help you easily reach your goals whether it be to lose weight, gain muscle, or just maintain better health. How about increasing your energy levels to feel unstoppable! Who doesn't want that?

It really comes down to understanding just three key things, what I refer to as SimpleSolutions, and these alone can change your life: master your mindset, nail your nutrition, and fit in fitness.

It's. So. Simple! Yet hardly anyone in pharmacy understands it because we don't teach it. It's barely taught in U.S. schools. Some of our friends and family may understand one or two pieces of it, but few fully understand the science behind it.

For me to truly grasp it feels like a gift I need to share. Others can become empowered and live life on their own terms while feeling amazing and actually enjoying the process along the way! To me, being a pharmacist is one of the most important things in my life. The relationships I have formed with my colleagues and patients through that trust is truly sacred. But being able to go even deeper and help people through nutrition is indescribable. I can help them really understand how to eat to reach their own goals by simplifying the science. It's really hard to put that gift into words, even for me!

> *"If you don't make time for your wellness,*
> *you will be forced to make time for your illness."*
> —Dr. Adam Martin

Now it's time to put self-care into action...

You've likely studied migraines and pain control in pharmacy school. If not, you will learn one of the most important counseling points that apply to both: do not wait for the pain to get super high before you decide to act and treat it. It takes far more to reduce high levels of pain than it would have if you treated (or acted) the moment you started to notice it escalate. The same concept is true for your own daily health and wellness. This is all summed up perfectly in this proverb by Benjamin Franklin:

> *"An ounce of prevention is worth a pound of cure."*

We all have the same twenty-four hours in a day—even Beyoncé has the time! It's not about *finding* time, it's about *making* time. Here's the truth:

> *If it's a priority, you'll make it happen.*
> *If it's not, you'll make an excuse.*

This is true, not just for your own self-care, but for everything you choose to do, or not do, in your life. This may be a hard pill to swallow (yeah, I said it) but the next time you say:

> *I don't have time for* ____
> replace that with:
> ____ *is not a priority.*
> and see how that feels.
> That will likely shift your perspective and lead
> to some changes in your (in)actions.

I want you to be able to eat for the rest of your life, to become your own best nutritionist. Using these SimpleSolutions, you can be at any pharmacy, hospital, medical school—anywhere in the world—and live healthily. My goal is to take the frustration out of nutrition and teach you to be in total control of what's going on in your body. You don't have to be a pharmacist, nutritionist, or anyone other than yourself—you just need a genuine desire to live life on your terms by controlling the controllables. With these SimpleSolutions, you can script your own success and live your ideal life of health. And *that* is what healthcare is all about—caring enough to lead others to optimal health.

This concept of self-care is so important to empower you to become not only the best pharmacist, but the best person you can be, that you could write an entire book on that concept alone! In fact, I did! It was my first book, titled R$_x$: *YOU! The Pharmacist's Survival Guide for Managing Stress & Fitting in Fitness*. If you want to take action, prioritize self-care, and make the most out of you, I strongly encourage you to pick up a copy. It's available online on Amazon in print and on Kindle for your convenience. Let me share the premise of that book and the path that led to it.

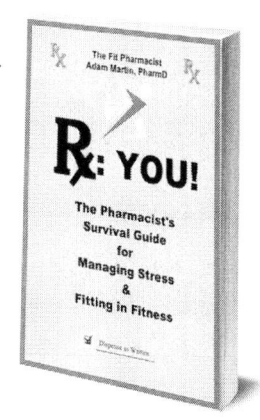

When I first embarked on my own fitness journey more than fifteen years ago, I was surprised by the results. Colleagues began asking me for tips, tricks, and recommendations they could use to feel healthy and look better. This struck a chord for me, as my main reason for becoming a pharmacist was to help people live healthier lives, but then it hit me: *who else serves patients?* Not just pharmacists, but phenomenal nurses, compassionate physicians, physician's assistants, and all of the other amazing professionals that are part of the healthcare team.

I began to connect with others in my profession who had overcome their own struggles in their journey toward health, and we began to share what we learned along the way. Those who were looking for a place to start improving their health became inspired and put that into action to actually become healthier and create a lifestyle to which they could adhere. This was the beginning of The Fit Pharmacist movement. It has grown far beyond what I could have ever imagined, inspiring and positively impacting the lives of not just pharmacists and pharmacy students, but nurses, PA's, physicians, and other healthcare professionals. It has begun to bridge the gap among practitioners, allowing us to relate to, support, and motivate each other to stick to our commitment to health, not just in our professional practice, but in our own daily lives.

This led to *The Fit Pharmacist Healthcare Podcast*, which is a source of weekly knowledge nuggets to aid in your pursuit of consistent and never-ending improvement—be sure to subscribe so you don't miss a single episode! The community that has been created by these amazing individuals continues to grow daily, and I am so proud to be a part of it. Our healthcare system has challenges. Some say it is in a crisis. Let's do our part to fix it. We must make it our mission to lead by example, to put health back into priority and be the change we wish to see across healthcare in our community. It all starts with us. I want to conclude this chapter by challenging you to ask yourself these questions:

EXERCISE

Write down your answers to the following questions, focusing on the first thing that comes to mind for each:

What is an area of my health that needs improvement?

_____

_____

_____

_____

_____

_____

_____

_____

Looking at mindset, nutrition, and physical fitness, is there one, two, or all three where I could be more skilled? Circle your answer(s).

   Mindset   Nutrition   Physical Fitness

Which ONE do I feel would best serve my professional and personal goals in the stage of life I am in right now? Circle your answer.

   Mindset   Nutrition   Physical Fitness

If I took action toward becoming more skilled in that area, how would I feel knowing that I am taking action toward improving myself in that one area?

_____

_____

_____

_____

_____

_____

_____

_____

By taking immediate action on improving my _____ , I would feel:

_____

_____

_____

_____

_____

_____

_____

_____

Finally, write this out as an act of service for you:

I AM WORTH IT!

(Go ahead: physically write it out below as big and bold as you want! This page belongs to you!)

It's not about *having* time—it's about *making* time. Make time work for you rather than being a slave to the clock. At times (pun), even if you follow all of the preceding advice, you may feel stuck, lost, overwhelmed, or even like you're drowning in tasks. If this is you, the next chapter will give you a script for the clarity and progress you've been looking for—that of practicing deep work.

Chapter 4

TAME TIME MANAGEMENT WITH DEEP WORK

"Time management is life management."

—Robin Sharma

WE ALL KNOW that one person who seems to have mastered the art of having more time than us. You know who I mean. The person who gets it all done, who's an energizer bunny when it comes to cranking out results, *and* seems to have more free time than us, *and* has more projects in their future than we can handle in our present, *and* has fun, making it look easy while they crush it! HOW? If we all have the same twenty-four hours in a day, what superpower does this magician have, and what spell do we have to cast in order to get it?

The secret is *deep work*. Those who fit the description of the unicorn described above may or may not have heard of this term, but I can guarantee you, that is how they are able to accomplish everything they do in the same amount of time that we all have. I first heard of deep work from author Cal Newport, who literally wrote the book, *Deep Work*, which I highly recommend adding to your reading list. Newport made some excellent points as it relates to dominating your time in pharmacy school. The first focuses on the biggest weakness of our generation: *patience*.

With the rise of reliance on technology, immediate gratification and innumerable distractions savage our attention—there always seems to be something new and exciting, every second! Think about it. When was the last time you were able to focus on one, and only one, task for one solid hour? No texting, checking social media, your email, or replying to a DM "just real quick"? It's hard to do it, #realtalk now. But if you succumb to the temptation to scroll through your feed or glance at your phone notifications, it will become much more difficult to complete whatever task you are trying to accomplish.

I'm not telling you to throw your phone away, or suggesting that you never use social media (how else would you be able to follow @thefitpharmacist on Instagram?), but I *am* telling you to be conscious of your environment. Can you see how all of these distractions vying for our valuable attention can wreak havoc on our level of focus and productivity? In our current culture, deep work is both rare and valuable. It's pretty difficult to accomplish with all these distraction, but if you can crack the code and commit to the practice of deep work, it will set you far above your competition and lead to levels of productivity that are unparalleled and effective. Your colleagues will wonder how you're crushing it!

As a testimony to the effectiveness of deep work, the second half of this book contains invaluable interviews with key professionals who have worked to become pioneers and experts in their respective niche of pharmacy practice. Each and every one of them perform deep work. It's no coincidence that these are related! Each interviewee was asked how they came to practice deep work so that *you* can learn from their process and get some ideas on how to adopt and practically apply this skill into your own lifestyle to empower you to dispense your full potential in both your professional and personal lives. Who better to learn this concept from than the best in our industry? I have compiled all of them right here in this book for you, my friend, so that you can spend time on your own deep work to maximize your pharmacy school experience!

> But, Adam, I have to work eighteen hours a day to really make big strides and have impact. That's not even a possibility as a pharmacy student with the workload I have, so what's the point in trying that now?

No! Research shows that four hours is the limit for how much deep work a human can do in one day. Backing this up are numerous examples of successful people who only put in four hours of deep work per day. One modern example is Andy Frisella, host of the number one business and entrepreneur podcast in the world as of this writing, the MFCEO Project. He practices and preaches what he describes as the Power List to start your day, in which you write down just five tasks to execute, not ten, not twenty—only five. He states that once those five items are complete, you have won the day and can proceed with doing other fun things, like being social and having family time—you know, living!

So, if you thought that you need to do double digit hours of deep work per day, you do not have to feel guilty anymore about the amount of actual work you get done each day. But, if you're checking social media during your deep work sessions, that attentional residue will add up rather quickly, and before you know it you will need to spend ten+ hours with that scattered work ethic to get the same amount of work done. Do you see that, by doing this, you can control time rather than feel like time controls you? Do the deep work, then go out and play all day. Sounds like an R_x4Success to me, FitPharmFam!

Now that we have gained some insight into *what* deep work is, let's dive into the really good part: *how* to put this magic incantation into practice!

Here are some action steps you can take paired with some SimpleSolutions to begin forming your deep work routine and strengthening your quality of productivity:

5 Steps to Develop Your Deep Work Habit

1. Figure out what is most valuable to your success. If you're having trouble with narrowing down to one thing, see the Resources section at the end for a resource recommendation to help you discover it.

2. Spend a scheduled amount of your time on that, *especially in the early hours of your day* when your attention span is stronger compared to the end of your day.

3. Aim to spend at least three deep sessions a day on your one thing. For each session, strive for a maximum of ninety-minute durations. You can start with smaller chunks of twenty or thirty minutes in the beginning until you form a habit. Building consistency into your daily rituals is your number one goal to start.

4. Almost anything other than your main task is considered a shallow task (e.g., social media or responding to emails). Recognize where you have been spending your time by identifying what your shallow tasks are and be sure to not engage with them during your allotted deep work timeframe.

5. Bunch all of your shallow tasks together into one deep task and set time aside for them. Knock them out in your schedule rather than being distracted by them all day!

Now you have a plan to create a deep work habit in five easy steps. As a future pharmacist, counting by five's will be your counting method of choice, so we are simultaneously building that skill and practice. How about that!

> But, Adam, how do I get more focused so that I can stay on task during my deep work session?

I gotchu, FitPharmFam! Often times, it's what we do outside of deep work sessions that sets us up to be more focused once the time for deep work comes. It's similar to stress management. In the moment of a stressful situation, it can be tricky to ease your anxiety if you haven't been practicing mindfulness and other ways to feel calm as a daily ritual outside of stressful situations. Here are some simple activities you can consider to help you strengthen your focus muscle:

Take a Walk

One simple action you can take to really invigorate your ability to focus on deep work is spending time in nature. No, I'm not saying you need to become Henry David Thoreau, but leave your technology behind and just go on a simple walk with the sole goal of noticing what you see. Take in the sights of the trees, the sounds of the birds singing, the feel of the wind on your face, the smell of the flowers—really put all of your focus into engaging as many of your senses as you can to really live in the moment.

This experience does not even have to be lengthy. You can start with just a half-hour leisurely stroll every week or two, or even a one-minute break just to refocus. The key is to make this a *consistent* dedication in your schedule, whatever you can realistically commit to on an ongoing basis *no matter what*. This may sound a bit strange at first, but trust me, coming from someone who used to be scatterbrained and who felt like my days were spent running around trying to put out fires, this simple trick will work wonders for your depth of focus, anxiety, productivity levels, and overall wellbeing.

Log Off

How many times per day do you check your email, social media notifications, or favorite websites? Shoot, how many times per hour do you find yourself mindlessly doing this out of habit, like a knee-jerk reaction? This may seem like a simple I'll-just-check-real-quick action, but the effect this has on your deep work tasks lasts much longer. It hinders your progress and sets you back roughly ten times the length of time it took you to check that Facebook post. This phenomenon is known as *attentional residue*. When it comes to technology and distractions overall, those glances and swipes cost you dearly in your productivity levels and are the number one killer to getting your tasks done efficiently.

The most rewarding and simple action step I've taken that has had the most profound impact on the quality of my deep work was a new habit I added during my morning rituals.

When I wake up in the morning, I commit to not checking my phone for at least two hours. Yes, the world will still be there, I promise you! Specifically, I plug my phone in to charge far away from my work area with the notifications off and in airplane mode.

But, Adam, I have to check_____.

And you can, after some deep work.

Sign Off

Knowing when to call it quits and sticking to it is almost as important as the deep work itself when it comes to long-term consistency in your productivity. You don't want to be a one-hit-wonder with your impact—you want this to last forever as you improve and grow each and every day.

Set a cutoff point each day and commit to calling it quits when that time arrives. Your brain needs to recharge. I've noticed that being "constantly on" really stresses me out and makes me less productive. Don't spend your relaxation time worrying about what needs to be done—that's not relaxing at all! Set it and forget it.

To end your day, create a shutdown ritual. This will serve two purposes: you'll be able to make sure there's nothing urgent left to do, and by doing this, you'll organize your tasks. Carrying out your shutdown ritual will signal to your mind to not be worried that it shut down too early and needs to get back to work. Link this habit to telling yourself that, yes, it's time for Mr. Sandman to work his magic, and, yes, you have permission to shift your focus to rest and recovery. Sweet dreams!

EXERCISE:

1. Identify **when** you can consistently commit to your deep work time (e.g., for the first sixty minutes of every morning, I will commit to my deep work).

   I can, I will, and I MUST consistently commit to _____ minutes of deep work at these times:

   _____

   _____

   _____

   _____

   _____

   _____

   _____

2. List out shallow work activities that you find yourself engaging in on a daily basis that distract you from your deep work (e.g., Instagram scrolling and checking emails).

   Shallow work activities I can bundle together and schedule for these times:

   _____

   _____

   _____

3. Identify simple activities you can adopt into your routine to improve your quality of focus (e.g., I will start each morning by walking for ten minutes).

A simple activity to increase my quality of focus that I can implement into my daily routine is:

4. Create your shutdown ritual to end every day. You will need to pick a shut down time and simple activities that can trigger your brain to recognize this as your end-of-day time to wind down and leave your worries behind (e.g., my shutdown time is 10PM, and I will trigger this by brushing my teeth).

I will designate my shut down time as ____ PM. My shut down ritual will begin by the simple act(s) of:

_____

_____

_____

_____

_____

_____

_____

Often, when pursuing a big goal or chasing your dream, you can feel alone, overwhelmed, or just lost. Hear me loud and clear, FitPharmFam, and know these truths: you are *not* alone and you do not have to go through what you're going through alone, either! As Najwa Zebian so eloquently said:

> *"These mountains that you are carrying,*
> *you were only supposed to climb."*

That is why if you ever do feel alone, overwhelmed, or at a loss for answers, it's essential that you (onward to the next chapter)...

Chapter 5

ASK FOR HELP PRN

"If you want to go fast, go alone; if you want to go far, go together."

—African Proverb

PRIDE IS SOMETHING that can literally destroy you. Please heed this advice if you ever find yourself in a tough spot slipping in your studies, grades, performance, networking, or professional responsibilities:

You do not have to go through it alone!

My goal is to empower your quest but it should not serve as a substitute for the irreplaceable value of face-to-face interaction with a professional at your specific institution. While there is variability in pharmacy schools, each one has a student resource center, pharmacy student community, or mentor program. Utilize this early on—*from or before day one!* You may not need it now, but one piece of advice that has served me well in life, especially when it came to pharmacy school, was from a banner that was on my 9th grade classroom wall:

"Today's preparation determines tomorrow's achievement."

Said in the context of the pharmacy world,

> *"An ounce of prevention is worth a pound of cure."*
> —Benjamin Franklin

There it is again! It must be something you should take seriously, if you're seeing it in this book twice!

This ties into the concept we will cover in a later chapter on creating a strong network for yourself: your network is your net worth. Expand that network by setting up a meeting with the director of your student resource center. That's literally what they're there for, to be a resource to help you! Again, you may not *need it* now, but lay the groundwork and set up that connection. Later down the road, when you feel like adding just one more thing to your plate would break you—like, say, setting up a meeting with the student resource center—you will have already taken care of that step!

> But, Adam, I am doing fine on my own right now—this advice doesn't apply to me.

I implore you, please, *please* take this advice seriously. Set your pride aside and set up a simple introductory meeting. Learn about the resources available, maybe not just for you, but perhaps for a friend in need who didn't read this book and gets in a tough spot down the road.

Within pharmacy school, there are so many amazing groups to not only foster your professional growth and development, but to network with the go-getters of your class, not to mention go-getters from other schools if you decide to attend regional and national conferences that many of the student pharmacist organizations offer every year. I was highly involved in Phi Delta Chi (PDC), the Student National Pharmaceutical Association (SNPhA), Phi Lambda Sigma (PLS), and served as the president of my class. All of these were so rewarding in my own development and added such a richness to my professional and personal life, that I am still good friends with many of those whom I met through being involved as a student. I went from being rejected from even getting into pharmacy school to writing this book on mastering pharmacy school that you are now holding in your hand. Getting involved in organizations and asking for help when I needed it seemed to work pretty well for me, and I *know* it will serve you well too!

Drug & Alcohol Abuse and Counseling

Yes, this does happen in pharmacy school. Stress can feel so suffocating at times, and create so much pain, that we just want it to stop. Life's burdens can feel so overwhelming that some turn to alcohol or other substances to cope. These choices jeopardize not only their health, but their professional careers. There are people in your life who care deeply about you! Don't believe me?

Consider this: there were hundreds, if not thousands, of potential pharmacy students who applied to your pharmacy school, and the administration and admissions committee chose *you*! Many students got declined during the application process, but the school chose *you*! That has to mean something! So, if you find yourself in a tough spot, know that we all go through them, and resources are available to help! People, groups, and professionals are available who specialize in *helping you*—not judging, not shaming, but guiding. *Make the call*—you are worth it!

If you or someone you care about is going through a tough time right now, please reach out to your student advisor, mentor, professor, or student center. In addition, here are some resources, which are by no means all-inclusive, for reaching professionals who can help you, a friend, loved one, or patient (*you can print a PDF copy of the following resources to post in your pharmacy at thefitpharmacist. com/resources*):

SAMHSA (Substance Abuse and Mental Health Services Administration)'s mission is to reduce the impact of substance abuse and mental illness on America's communities.

National Helpline: 1-800-662-HELP (4357)
Website: www.samhsa.gov/find-help/national-helpline
"This helpline provides 24-hour free and confidential treatment referral and information about mental and/or substance use disorders, prevention, and recovery in English and Spanish."

Disaster Distress Helpline: 1-800-985-5990
Website: www.samhsa.gov/find-help/disaster-distress-helpline
"Stress, anxiety, and other depression-like symptoms are common reactions after any natural or human-caused disaster. Call this toll-free number to be connected to the nearest crisis center for information, support, and counseling."

Suicide Prevention Lifeline: 1-800-273-TALK (8255)
Website: www.suicidepreventionlifeline.org
"24-hour, toll-free, confidential suicide prevention hotline available to anyone in suicidal crisis or emotional distress. Your call is routed to the nearest crisis center in the national network of more than 150 crisis centers."

Veteran's Crisis Line: 1-800-273-TALK (8255)
Website: www.veteranscrisisline.net
"Connects veterans in crisis (and their families and friends) with qualified, caring Department of Veterans Affairs responders through a confidential, toll-free hotline, online chat, or text."

Behavioral Health Treatment Services Locator
Website: www.findtreatment.samhsa.gov
"Find alcohol, drug, or mental health treatment facilities and programs around the country."

Buprenorphine Physician & Treatment Program Locator
Website: www.samhsa.gov/medication-assisted-treatment/physician-program-data/treatment-physician-locator
"Find information on locating physicians and treatment programs authorized to treat opioids, such as heroin or prescription pain relievers."

Early Serious Mental Illness Treatment Locator
Website: www.samhsa.gov/esmi-treatment-locator
"Find treatment programs in your state that treat recent onset of serious mental illnesses such as psychosis, schizophrenia, bi-polar disorder, and other conditions."

Opioid Treatment Program Directory
Website: https://dpt2.samhsa.gov/treatment/
"Find treatment programs in your state that treat addiction and dependence on opioids, such as heroin, or prescription pain relievers."

Poison Control Center: 1-800-222-1222
Text POISON to 797979 to save the contact info for poison control in your phone
Website: www.poisonhelp.org
"Poison control centers offer free, confidential, expert medical advice 24/7."
Life-Threatening Emergency: 9-1-1

Yes, it's true that *a smooth sea never made a skilled sailor*, but when you're in the middle of a hurricane, it's much more helpful to let the crew on deck help you rather than trying to manage everything by yourself. Sounds silly, right?

Speaking of being out at sea, perhaps you not only love pharmacy, but sailing, too! There's a reason I brought a seemingly unrelated hobby like sailing into this book on pharmacy school. There is inherent value in having a passion outside of your pharmacy career. *Having a non-pharmacy hobby can make or break your long-term success as a pharmacist.* Does that sound counterintuitive? Allow me to explain...

Chapter 6

THE VALUE OF AN OUTSIDE PASSION

"When one door closes, another opens; but we often look so long and so regretfully upon the closed door that we do not see the one which has opened for us."

—Alexander Graham Bell

YOU'VE LIKELY HEARD the advice to *go all in* on one and only one thing. It makes sense to stay focused on one initiative. I have learned something different from numerous pharmacists at the top of their respective fields. In fact, once I began expanding hobbies, I found that it served me well both in my personal and professional life.

> But, Adam, I want to be excellent in pharmacy—if I try to do other things, I'll just spread myself too thin!

First, let me ask you a question. Have you ever been in the middle of writing a paper, working on a really big project, or maybe even writing a book (meta right there), and just felt like your eyes were glazing over? That your level of productivity was dropping faster than Tessalon Perles® flying off the counting tray into the abyss of the amber vial bin?

Let's start with another question. What's the feeling you had in that moment of writer's block?

I need a fresh set of eyes!

I need a break!

I need to just talk a walk!

%&^@$*#!!!!!!!*

Yes, to all of the above! Taking a break, like ten minutes for every fifty minutes of work, can be a useful tactic to prevent burnout in the short term, but what about the long-term game? What about the bigger picture—your career?

I am fascinated by those in our profession who are literally the best at what they do, those who go far beyond their colleagues in terms of passion and productivity. In meeting these professionals, I have sought to learn how they are able to perform at such a high level for extended periods of time. One thing I consistently noticed in almost all of their lives was an outside passion, some activity or interest *not* directly related to their career.

It was intriguing to see pharmacists, not only the absolute best at what they did in their careers, but who were also good at some other thing, whether an exceptional cook, whiskey connoisseur, race car driver, MMA fighter, or fitness fanatic. The more high-performing professionals that I met, the more I realized that having an outside hobby was like a blueprint for achieving excellence. That's why I dedicated an entire chapter of this book to recommend this to you, as a future pharmacist. You can use it to craft your own version of greatness and have the assurance knowing your side hobby, passion project, or guilty pleasure will serve you well in both your pharmacy career and overall quality of life for two reasons.

A hobby outside of your career helps prevent burnout, one of the most common career killers in our profession. Life is meant to be lived, so find that special activity that really gets you excited and giddy when you think about it! For me, that's physical fitness, and just typing that out makes me smile. So go find your smile-maker!

You will also likely experience a form of skill transfer that will help you solve problems and innovate or increase your productivity in ways you may not have considered. Allow me to explain what I mean.

Have you ever been stuck on a project, and someone said to you, *we just need to approach this from a different angle*? If you keep trying to solve a problem using the same method of thinking that you've been using, do you think anything different will result? A wise guy once said,

> *"Insanity is doing the same thing over and over and expecting different results"*

It was Einstein, that wise guy. This is one reason why interprofessional collaboration, especially in healthcare, is so valuable in addressing some of the biggest issues we are trying to solve. Each profession is trained in a different way unique to crafting their skills. Tremendous insight comes from overlap and working in an area that is similar but different. This allows a fresh set of eyes to consider how to solve the problem using a totally different approach.

When one door closes, another opens—you've likely heard this before. What if instead of just another door, something else opens, something that was not initially even considered? If you keep this in mind, and look to not think outside the box, but rather away from the door, you may just be met with a window of opportunity.

EXERCISE

Write down a hobby or activity that you enjoy outside of ClubPharmacy. Something that when you do or think about doing it, you become excited and full of energy and anticipation. In addition, write down **why** you like it (**e.g., I love to work out because it makes me feel amazing, is an investment in my overall health, and teaches me the principles of delayed gratification, the value of hard work, and personal accountability**).

My favorite non-pharmacy-related activity is:

_____

_____

_____

_____

_____

I love to _____ **because:**

_____

_____

_____

_____

_____

_____

> **If you have not yet found your ideal activity, rephrase the above with:**
>
> My favorite non-pharmacy-related activity
> I would like to pursue is:
>
> And
>
> I would love to _____ because:
>
> _____
> _____
> _____
> _____
> _____
> _____

As you can see, it's always good to have a *my thing* type of hobby or passion. Once you give yourself permission to fully embrace you as you, and do those things that truly make you happy and fulfilled, this emotion of self-realization will create clarity for your passion. This will give you ultimate personal power as you are being genuinely authentic to who you are and what really invigorates you to forge your personal and professional identity and goals! This will ultimately lead you to create your own *personal brand*.

Chapter 7

BUILDING YOUR PERSONAL BRAND AND YOUR COMPETITIVE EDGE

*"Your brand is what people say about you
when you are not in the room."*

—Jeff Bezos, founder of Amazon®

YOU ARE NOW in pharmacy school—WOOHOO! While you may be focused on studying pharmacy, I am going to share a secret with you. If you want to really excel in our profession, you'll need to learn some basics about business.

That's right. I am about to share with you one concept taught in business that will empower you to excel in pharmacy at a level that sets you far beyond those who do not practice this.

> But, Adam, I am studying to become a pharmacist!
> I don't have any interest in the business side of the profession.
> I'm not looking to own my own pharmacy—I just
> want to focus on learning pharmacy and help
> my patients the very best way that I can!

If you want to make a big impact, you must realize one truth. The key to success in our profession hinges on one main focus: *relationships*. If you can learn to master this concept, it will position you to serve your patients on a much deeper level, setting you up for constant and never-ending improvement in your skills and abilities not just as a pharmacist, but as a person. You will see continual growth and increased levels of impact. Who doesn't want that!

In pharmacy school, we face many demands. We study, join student organizations, complete projects, pass exams... oh, yeah, and class! But if that is all we do, we will just be the same as everyone else who gets a PharmD. Don't get me wrong, pharmacy school was one of the best times of my life and I have tremendous respect and loyalty for my alma mater. However, if we set the nostalgia aside and look at this from a business perspective, how will you make yourself unique? How will you stand above the crowd and offer something extra so that when it comes to job interviews, you provide so much value that you are an easy candidate to *immediately* favor?

What if the head honchos at the pharmacy you are applying at already knew you ahead of time and smiled as soon as they saw you because you had put in the effort and time to make that connection? What if you went above and beyond to foster your first encounter into a cordial relationship by following up, thus demonstrating your work ethic? Would it be just a friendly hello, or would you leave the impression that there is something special about you—something extra that makes them think, *there's just something about this one I really like!*

You won't create any clout in the library or from your couch— you have to go out into the marketplace and market yourself! Yes, I said market yourself, as in developing your own *personal brand.* Who are you? What do you represent? What are you super passionate about, to the point that when you start talking about it, your genuine enthusiasm gets other people excited as well?

That is what it takes in this competitive economy we know as pharmacy! It doesn't matter what niche you're pursuing, with what company you're seeking employment, or what post-graduate studies you're hoping to continue, *how you brand and market yourself makes the difference!*

This might seem a little intimidating, maybe even a little overwhelming to say the least.

> But, Adam, you mean to tell me that on top of my schoolwork and class time and projects and exam prep—I need to do more?

No. I am *imploring* you to make the most of your potential by setting yourself up as a positive influence and doing what you really love! Now is the time. Waiting will only give your competition time to seize your space and build a stronger presence. Don't you want to be the go-to expert in something which you're extremely passionate? How would that make you feel? Pretty pumped and grateful, right?

There are five things to consider when you embark on representing yourself as a brand in order to embody your message and mission as effectively as possible to your audience:

- Quality content
- Consistency
- Congruency
- Innovation
- Collaboration

If you want to make an impact with something that's important to you, where do you even start? You've put in the work to learn your craft and are committed to develop mastery, but how can you elevate your reach? Relationships! You need to meet people with genuine intentions to give and serve rather than receive.

For an example of this as an action, let's turn to the world of social media. If you have a LinkedIn® profile, you know that it focuses on one main thing: relationships. The connections we have in our personal and professional lives link us into their networks, and we share those as a means to collaborate, grow, learn, and prosper.

If you use LinkedIn®, perhaps you have heard of the most successful user of this platform, Lewis Howes. This man was a professional football player who experienced a stop to his career from an injury, leaving him unemployed, living on his sister's couch, and gifted with time to figure out what to do with his life. From perceived failure came outstanding opportunity, and through a chain of events, Lewis was led to LinkedIn®. He used this platform to not only make some serious professional connections, but create his career and personal brand!

I had the pleasure of attending the 2018 10X Growth Conference where he was one of the guest speakers. The message he delivered was very clear: *build a massive audience and pump up your personal brand!* Lewis gave a call to action to not just live our lives, but to build our brands around our dreams and *truly* live!

As he shared the genesis of his own personal brand, he spoke about the event of 2009 when "everything changed for me."

The talk he delivered was titled "My Sweaty Pits and A Cat Named Leaf Moose," referring to his sister's cat, who he described as "a fat, hairy, unsocial, and just nasty cat." Lewis said the cat didn't like people, and especially did not get along with him. Despite this relationship, the cat had a place in Lewis's start towards professional growth.

As he continued to consistently provide valuable content and network on the platform, Lewis soon became known as "the LinkedIn guy." This led to an opportunity for him to join a webinar to teach some of his skills and share the knowledge he had developed on LinkedIn. He explained that, at the time, he had no real presentation skills or know-how regarding webinars or leveraging in the sales space, so he just got online and spoke about what he knew. He made a decision to offer one of his information products for sale. At the conclusion of the webinar, in which he invested one hour of his time, he ended up making $6,200. He was so excited at the unexpected positive response that he grabbed the only thing around him at the time, the dirty cat Leaf Moose, and embraced him wholeheartedly, despite the cat's hiss of refusal. His point: "If I can make $6,200 in one hour while being sweaty with a nasty cat in my sister's house, I can scale this out!"

Initially, Lewis considered relying on selling other people's products as an affiliate. However, he quickly realized that this approach was unsustainable, and that he needed a defined personal brand. He reached a conclusion that shaped the course of his future, career, and life mission: "If you want scalable sales, you've got to invest in your personal brand and offer consistent value to build a massive audience!"

This might sound like a huge task, especially if you haven't considered yourself to be a personal brand before. The first thing you must ask yourself as you embark on your journey is *what is my message to the world?* For Lewis, it revolved around gratitude. This led him to partner with a non-profit organization called Pencils of Promise, which aims to increase children's access to quality education.

Once he found his message, he set out to share it with his audience and the world through the medium of podcasting. This he scaled through three main actions:

- Building a personal brand
- Adding value
- Building a massive audience

Building a brand takes time. Be patient and be consistent. Engagement, subscribers, and growth are some key indicators, ones that Lewis has shown are effective.

Looking at the growth of these three indicators of his social media platforms, he seems to know what he's doing:

Podcasting Downloads: 2013: 770,000; 2014: 53 MIL

Instagram Followers: 2016: 95,000; 2017: 276,000; 2018: 620,000

Lewis gave one main piece of advice to achieve a growth trajectory like this: *constantly reinvest into your personal brand.* You will increase your reach if you increase your audience and relationship conversion.

Personal brand + mass audience = 10X Growth

Engagement is a key area of focus that Lewis defined as a successful keystone quality for growing a personal brand.

> *"Responding [to comments/engagement outreach] builds a relationship that resonates with the audience and connects with people."*

Lewis then went on to define what he labels as:

5 Keys to Building Your Personal Brand and Mass Audience:

1. Relationships

If you focus on investing in people, you will find allies that are more resourceful than you. Focus on one thing: *value.* What do you bring to the table? If you are in it for yourself in a *gimme-this* mindset, people will pick up on that and won't want to engage with you. Focus on giving from a genuine place. Everyone wins when you give.

2. Consistent Content

There are so many people, things, and businesses vying for our attention, so if we are going to commit to one avenue, we expect some level of commitment back. Build a schedule to which you can regularly adhere on an almost religious basis to build brand loyalty. Ensure consistent delivery of content to your audience. People love routine and someone on whom they can rely. *You* can be that person and brand! Do something unique that adds value to something about which you are passionate. Hosting interviews with key people in your area of interest is a great way to build a mass audience in your field. Create or add to your community and they will see your value!

3. Promotion and Press

If you are consistently in the news with key influencers in your area of expertise, seen over and over, people won't be able to miss you! Keep that up while creating consistent value and soon you be become *So Good They Can't Ignore You.*

4. Epic Design & Branding

By literally branding yourself with an image, logo, or the aesthetic feel of presence, you will grow and build from your brand identity. Lewis learned this early on when he approached a television network with which he wanted to collaborate. They turned him down. "Just by taking one look at your website, we'd never have you on the show." What a wake-up call! Lesson learned.

5. Unique Product

To stand out as valuable, present your brand as just a little bit different. The example Lewis gave was his latest book, *Mask of Masculinity*, spoke about men being vulnerable. At the time, no one was marketing vulnerability, so Lewis decided to use this open space as an opportunity to provide a resource that would allow men to drop their masks and be vulnerable. Novel idea, right?

The main question you need to ask yourself when trying to create a brand is *what image am I going to create that's different from anything similar in its space?* Find an answer that provides something that stands out and is unique.

Finding the right people to support your mission is a huge key to long-term success. Massive action requires a team, and finding the right players is essential to having a massive impact on a massive audience. In order to build a legacy brand, start by identifying and creating just that: an audience. Pharmacy has a pretty huge audience, so how are you going to create your own personal brand? What one area of focus in pharmacy are you most passionate? Looking at the previous chapter, what was your one non-pharmacy hobby that you love? Identify the answer to each of these questions and pair those with your natural talents and abilities to find the right direction to create your very own personal brand to dispense the passion, purpose, and service of value to your audience.

EXERCISE:

We will look at three unique parts of you and then combine them to create your personal brand focus:

$$1 + 2 + 3 = R_x$$

Write down which area of pharmacy you are most interested, or drawn to, and why.

1. The area of pharmacy that I feel most drawn to is:

_____
_____
_____
_____
_____

I feel called to pursue this particular niche primarily because:

_____
_____
_____
_____
_____
_____

✛

Revisit the previous chapter on The Value of an Outside Passion and add your responses below.

2. My favorite non-pharmacy activity that I love is:

_____

_____

_____

_____

_____

_____

_____

_____

I love to _____ **because:**

_____

_____

_____

_____

_____

_____

_____

_____

+

Write down your natural talents and abilities below.

3. One of my gifts and talents that I have a natural tendency to be good at is:

_____

_____

_____

_____

_____

_____

_____

Now you have the three parts and can formulate your R_x:

=

R_x: My personal brand focus will be:

_____

_____

_____

_____

_____

_____

_____

You can't show up for others at your best if you don't first know and show up for yourself, as we discussed in the self-care chapter. Once you commit to that process, the level of clarity you gain from doing what you love will create your identity of service for others.

What you stand for, how you serve, plus your personal vision, is YOUR PERSONAL BRAND.

I just now mentioned the process to define this place of clarity, and a process it *is*! You will not wake up and say *AHA! I know exactly what I am going to do with my life!* This isn't something to groan about (remember patience and delayed gratification?), but something to celebrate, as you are embarking on a journey filled with never-ending growth and improvement—*that* is exciting! It's like pharmacy. Look at all of the changes that happen on a daily basis, some small, some large. Take a look at the profession five, ten, or twenty years ago and then look at the present day. Yes, prescriptions used to be kept with no computer entries at all—how? Imagine if it still operated that way today. This path of growth, innovation, and evolution seen in the profession is also what you should seek to create for yourself! It's change. It's innovation. It's discovering yourself on a deeper and deeper level so that you can better serve your patients, colleagues, friends, family, and yourself through the value you empower yourself to deliver.

We are all in different places in life. Self-awareness is essential to laying the groundwork for your journey. This is what is known as having *emotional intelligence*, one of the core character qualities we will now explore in creating your formula for ultimate success.

(R) RELATIONSHIP BUILDING

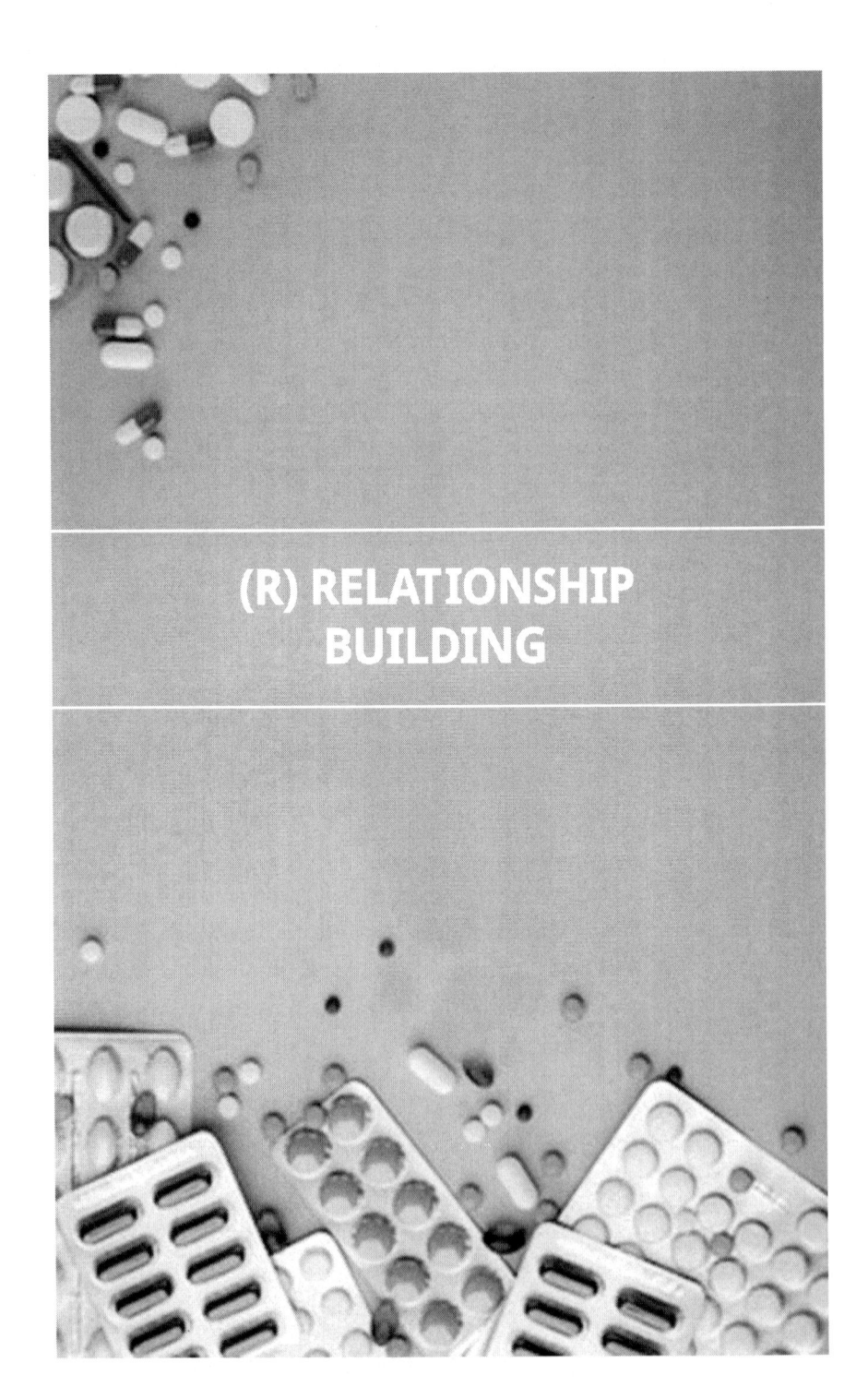

Chapter 8

MASTER YOUR EMOTIONAL INTELLIGENCE

"Mastering yourself is true power."

—Lao Tzu

AS A PHARMACIST, you will be helping people who, more often than not, are trying to improve their health. Whether it is an acute health crisis, initial burdensome diagnosis, or overwhelming co-morbid condition, this may be the most important focus they have. It could mean *their lives*. You will work with them directly, through counseling, navigating their insurance coverage, and ensuring proper adherence through medication therapy management.

> But, Adam, I am in pharmacy school to become a pharmacist—not a psychologist!

Many times, you will be with the patient, focused on their personal wellbeing. Emotions can range from anger, frustration, shame, remorse, loss of hope, disgust, sadness, or confusion. These are just some of the feelings that will be expressed, either *to* you or inadvertently *toward* you. How you handle the situation, and yourself, can mean the difference between building a patient relationship of trust, or of one lacking empathy. Which do you think will lead to better outcomes for those whom you serve as a pharmacist? The key to forming a healthy patient relationship hinges on what is known as *emotional intelligence.*

Perhaps you have heard the phrase emotional intelligence before, but what exactly *is* it? How do you become more emotionally intelligent? In this chapter, we will look at the five components of emotional intelligence as discussed by Harvard Psychologist Daniel Goleman in his 2001 book *Emotional Intelligence* and how you can increase this essential quality.

1. Part I: Self-Awareness
2. Part II: Self-Regulation
3. Part III: Motivation
4. Part IV: Empathy
5. Part V: Social Skill

Self-Awareness

What does it mean to be self-aware? Having the ability to know if you have spinach in your teeth without looking in the mirror? Perhaps a form of ESP about what you're going to do next? Or does it mean something more—something that can impact your relationships, leadership ability, and ability to build the best version of you? Let's take a look!

Self-awareness is developing a deep understanding of your emotions, needs, strengths, weaknesses, and motivations. This doesn't just come down to whether or not you are an introvert or extrovert in your social interactions, but rather your level of honesty with yourself and your peers in respect to the aforementioned qualities.

Let's look at an example of working in the pharmacy. You know you are going to have a short-staffed day, and that pressure really gets to you. You could plan ahead by calling someone to come in to help, or maybe leave earlier for your shift to get a head start on your work. In essence, cutting down your stress level *before* it begins.

We have all interacted with hot-tempered patients at one time or another. A pharmacist with a high level of self-awareness will be able to interact with this patient and maintain their cool. They will understand that the patient probably has more going on behind the scenes than meets the eye. Rather than falling victim to the temper, the pharmacist may even turn it into a positive interaction that benefits the patient—so much so that the patient will return for that excellent level of care received by the self-aware pharmacist and rave to their friends and family about *my* pharmacist.

The next component of self-awareness comes from your motives—your *recognition of values and goals*. Do you know what you are working toward, and *why* you want to end up there? A self-aware person will say yes (see why that was the first chapter?)!

If you really love working in a hospital setting, and want to build a practice alongside a physician, but are offered a high-paying job in a retail setting, your decision will reveal your level of self-awareness. Knowing *what* your passion and goals are and recognizing that this opportunity does not coincide with what's really important to you will likely lead you to pass on the offer.

If your values are reflected in your decisions, you are displaying self-awareness. Self-knowledge is invaluable to growing as a person. The ability to *admit your faults, own up to your actions, and learn from them to move forward* is what drives us to become better human beings. Seeking constructive criticism to improve yourself rather than ignoring helpful feedback is a common feature among the self-aware.

This ties closely with *self-confidence*—specifically knowing your strengths and aligning yourself to best utilize them. When you encounter a situation that engages your weaknesses, having the gusto to ask for help is seen as a display of strength rather than failure. If you've been reading this book in sequence, you have explored your strengths and interests in pharmacy to create your own personal brand, as well as recognized the value of setting pride aside to ask for help PRN.

Self-Regulation

Emotions, as I'm sure you know, riddle our everyday lives and can range about as much as the path of a roller coaster. That does not make us weak, just human! What can make us appear *super* human is our ability to control or *regulate* the normal emotions we experience.

In a single day, we can feel sad, happy, angry, excited, fearful—the list is endless! Having these feelings is normal; being a prisoner to them can wreak havoc in life.

Enter self-regulation: managing your emotions so that you can control them, and even use them to be constructive! When you are faced with an unexpected situation that evokes anger—a disaster at work, someone cutting you off on the road, or getting an unexpected bill in the mail—how do you react? Do you explode first then assess later? Or do you step back, look at the big picture and ask yourself *why did this happen?* Do you pause and think in order to find the best solution? The latter is an example of a strong sense of self-regulation, the former, not so much.

So, Adam, this is neat and all, but so what?
Why does this matter? What's the impact?

I think adopting the skill of self-regulation will positively impact your relationships, business, and overall life in three ways:

1. Being able to self-regulate will enable you to *create an environment of trust and fairness*. Being in control of your emotions helps avoid hurt and misunderstandings. People will be attracted to you, much like a Pittsburgher is drawn to a Stillers game (no, that's not a typo—that's how it's spelled n'at, yinzers). Taking this one step further, if you're in a leadership position, *you will set the standard.* If the boss is level-headed and fair, you'll look like quite the asshat if you're blowing up at the slightest sign of upset. Strong self-regulation in management will dissuade others from disrupting the peaceful mindset that is the status quo.

2. Change is inevitable. *Having a strong ability to self-regulate will allow you to adapt.* Speaking from the pharmacy world, where new medications are frequently added or taken off the market, laws are enforced, and recalls are announced, change is expected! I would say it's an *essential* skill in our profession.

3. Being able to avoid acting on impulse will prevent the pitfalls that are all too commonly seen on news headlines (e.g., executives involved in scandals). Where do these pitfalls begin? Impulsive behavior. When the chips are down, and you're not aware of your emotions, it can be very easy to act from desperation instead of logic. Focusing on the long-term win versus short-term gain can help you maintain perspective!

To recap, how can I tell if I have strong self-regulation skills?

1. Consider your and everyone's emotions before speaking.
2. Expect the unexpected and learn to adapt.
3. Avoid impulsive behavior.

Motivation

The one trait everyone wants more of—the cure-all people deem as the solution to their slump, the magic bullet to get things done—is *motivation*. Yes! One of the most inspiring qualities a leader can have is to consistently live their lives and carry out their work with a high sense of drive. The pure form of this does not come from *external* cues—materialistic drivers to perform—but *an intrinsic need to achieve for the sake of a deep purpose.*

There are signals you can use to detect and mark your level of motivation:

1. Passion

A deep love for the work you are doing cannot be faked. Ask yourself, *what really ignites my passion? What makes my eyes widen and smile broaden when someone just mentions the work/project/idea?* This level of intrigue in a passionate individual runs so deep that they will seek out challenges, have a thirst to learn, and find immense satisfaction in a job well done.

2. Raise the bar

Passion is also being *relentless* in your pursuit of excellence and never settling for the status quo, even if you have already redefined what that is in your prior successes. Did you hit your mark on your last project? Cross your T's and dot your I's? Nice! Next time, that won't be acceptable. Move the target. Stretch yourself to dispense your full potential knowing that you won't settle for an easy task. Raise the bar.

3. Set your target

Have you ever heard of SMART goals? These help motivated individual keep score as a means to track their progress along their path to achievement. You are putting in a lot of time, effort, and sweat, so you want to follow up along the way to make sure things are going according to plan. Many times, when your plan falls apart, be it from no fault of your own, you will have to be resilient. If setbacks or failures occur, the motivated individual will remain optimistic even when the odds are not in their favor. Rather than seeing it as a loss, instead the drawback is seen as an opportunity to prove it can be overcome. Looking at the previous pillars of emotional intelligence, we are pairing self-regulation with motivation to come out on top even when things aren't going our way.

And guess what? Things *never* go according to plan one hundred percent of the time, so this is a useful skill to develop to empower you through all the curveballs that life *will* send your way!

Looking at these components from a leadership perspective, if you are in a position of influence and you set these standards for yourself, you will do the same for those you lead. Why? Because all of these qualities are contagious! Maintaining a positive attitude and showing relentless commitment to the task at hand are non-negotiable in leading with success whether it's leading a team or your own life.

Empathy

In daily life, *empathy* is that warm quality we yearn for in our friends—that ability to listen to our worries and woes and to comfort us when we expose our true feelings of vulnerability. Yes, we love that friend! Shift this character trait to the business world and all of the sudden our perception of this changes. Hugs at work? Do we work at Snuggle®?

In business, the workplace, and leadership overall, empathy is often misunderstood as adopting others' feelings and working to make everyone happy. That, I can tell you, never works. So, then, what is it? Rather than acting on your own accord, acting with empathy means *to consider other people's feelings while making a judgment call*—to see it from their perspective.

Reflecting back on the leadership roles I served in throughout pharmacy school, and now as a pharmacist, has shown me how integral empathy is to becoming a higher-quality leader. Specifically, I've found three main reasons why this attribute is essential to your emotional intelligence repertoire:

1. **Teamwork**

    In order to make things happen, you need to work with people. You will always work with different *types* of people, regardless of your work environment, so expect different personality types! Along with that comes numerous different emotions in reaction to varying situations. Leading teams of people requires an acute *awareness* of these emotions, their implications, and the reasons behind them so that you can give voice to all the members of the team. Having a strong sense of empathy will enable you to more effectively navigate this variety. Do right by people and you shall do no wrong!

2. **Pace of globalization**

    A group of people from different backgrounds and cultures can lead to potential misinterpretations, varying levels of emotional sensitivities, and potential interpersonal catastrophes. The remedy for this challenge is empathy. A heightened sense of awareness of those things not directly spoken, like body language, enables you to read between the lines, affording you the opportunity to address issues before misunderstandings occur.

3. Keep talent on your team

Good help is hard to find. This is something we hear all too often in the work world. If you've ever worked in a pharmacy, you are likely aware of one of the golden rules of ClubPharmacy: a pharmacist is only as good as their tech, and a great tech is worth their weight in gold—and then some! Groom the best to be better and show genuine care to your team. This will result in better quality of care for your patients. Also important: be the talent others want to keep! It's a win-win-win across the board.

Social Skill

So far, we have looked at the first four components of emotional intelligence as individual factors. The fifth factor, *social skill*, ties all of these together into one cohesive ability to interact with others in such a way that you can foster relationships that position you to take massive action.

Hearing social skill at face value, you might think, *oh, piece of cake—I love social hour!*

Not so fast, sorority sister, there's more that meets the eye with this ability than just being sociable! It's more than just getting along with others. It's friendliness with a purpose—motivating people to come together and put their purpose into action.

The simplest way to depict this skill can be seen in high school cliques. The jocks, the nerds, the fashionistas—more often than not, these groups tend to stick with one another and not stray from the familiar. Then there are the independents—those who don't stick with one clique, but have friends from all the different circles. This is social skill at its finest, the ability to have a wide circle of acquaintances through finding commonalities.

How can you spot someone in action who displays strong social skills?

1. Someone who is skillful at managing teams (empathy)
2. Someone with a strong level of influence (self-awareness, self-regulation, and empathy combined)
3. Someone who inspires others through their enthusiasm for their purpose (motivation)

Leaders know that relationships need to be nurtured effectively in unison for one purpose. A whole unit moving together is greater than one person acting alone. What makes that plan turn into real action? Social skill! In simple terms, it is the vehicle that puts a leader's emotional intelligence to use for the good of the team.

We have talked about each of the five characteristics of emotional intelligence and how they all interrelate to yield effective action. Now the good news: emotional intelligence can be learned! You can develop the skill, much like you can grow and develop your muscles by lifting weights. However, just like workouts, it takes consistent dedication, effort, and time. Looking at the benefits of each section described in this chapter, it is worth it!

EXERCISE:

1. After reading the five core components of emotional intelligence, which ONE have you identified as an area you need to improve in your life?

The one component of emotional intelligence that I can most improve is:

_____

_____

_____

_____

_____

_____

_____

_____

2. What aspect of your daily life and interactions would improve if you worked to develop this skill?

If I work on developing my skill of _____ , my life and interactions would improve such that:

_____

_____

_____

In the beginning of this chapter, we discussed the importance of relationships for living a successful and fulfilled life. Particularly when building your personal brand, interacting with people in person is essential. The best place to do that in the context of pharmacy school is through *networking at conferences*. But how do you prepare for a conference? What are the best ways to network to make the most of your time? When it comes to following up with the new contacts you've made, what are you supposed to say without making it awkward or fake? So much to know—it can feel overwhelming! Not to worry, my friend, I've got you covered.

Chapter 9

NURTURE YOUR NETWORKING

"Your network is your net worth."

—Tim Sanders, former Yahoo!® Leadership Coach

IF YOU WANT to make an impact with something important to you, where do you start? You've put in the work to learn your craft and are committed to consistent improvements to develop your mastery, but how can you elevate your reach? Build intentional relationships!

It's especially true in the competitive market that pharmacy is today—*who you know* and *how you provide value to them* will be the ultimate leverage to open doors. Meeting people and presenting yourself as a valuable brand is the best thing you can do to make this happen. Live your mission.

> But, Adam, I have people to learn from already at my pharmacy school—why would I want to leave that comfort and convenience?

Wouldn't it be great to collaborate with a like-minded colleague on the same path as you? Or better yet, what if you could learn from someone who has already achieved what you plan to accomplish? What if I told you there is one place where all three groups of these people meet? Oh snap, son—it does exist!

No, it's not Narnia or Hogwarts (that's pharmacy school). It is, in fact, *conferences*! That's right, real-life people in a physical space with whom you can connect, meet in person, and even shake hands! There is tremendous value to online or summit-based web conferences, but you just can't replace in-person interaction.

Learning people skills only comes from building skills with people. You can read and rehearse all you want, but until you get in front of someone and make mistakes, perfect your pitch, and learn the nuances of nonverbal communication, you will never be a master. You must get in front of people—let's go!

If you've never been to a conference before, or it's been a very long time and was in a totally different arena (Boy Scouts summer camp perhaps?), you may feel a bit nervous, unprepared, and maybe even scared of what to expect. Good! That is a cue that you are headed in the right direction. I know that for two reasons:

1. The comfort zone is nice, but nothing every grows there.

2. If you are the smartest person in the room, you need to find a new room.

You should strive to move into unfamiliar territory with untapped potential. There, you can learn something new from those more advanced than you. Events create the big-ticket opportunities you need as a pharmacy student to grow your career. Increasing your confidence and effectiveness requires three elements:

1. Prep *before* the conference

2. Crush it *at* the conference

3. Focus on the *follow-up*

PART I: PREP BEFORE THE CONFERENCE

It's true: prior preparation prevents poor performance. Looking back at my time in pharmacy school, I feel blessed to say I ended up attending seven regional and national conferences, and I continue to attend them still to this day! I made a lot of mistakes and had some major, uh, "learning moments" over the years (that's a nice way to say epic fails). I want to share these moments with you now to set you up like a superhero with your R$_x$4Success. That way you can conquer any conference with confidence!

The Pharmacy Conference Fantastic Four:

1. Dress to Impress
2. Know Your Target
3. Fuel for Success
4. Sharp Body, Sharp Mind

Dress to Impress

When it comes to addressing (pun) the question of what to wear, there are two big mistakes I've seen pharmacy students make. Either they think they have to go over-the-top and buy an Armani suit/Gucci dress, or they say, *jeans are good, right?* Great news! Dressing professionally does not have to cost you an arm and a leg. I know firsthand about the financial burdens many face as pharmacy students. Consider these tips to help you elevate your style game without doing the same to your credit card debt:

- Join your favorite clothing store's email list for deals.
- Google "[store name] + coupon"—this works wonders!
- Use the website Honey® to autoscan any website for available coupons that will actually work (joinhoney.com/ref/1mxccl).
- Check out TJMaxx®, Marshalls®, or outlet malls (note: not recommended last minute!).
- Thrift stores like Goodwill® have amazing treasures at prices you wouldn't believe. Check them out—you never know what you'll find!

Know Your Target

Attend a conference with clear goals in mind to get the most out of your experience. Ask yourself what you want to get out of your trip.

Who do I want to meet while there?
What would I like to learn?
What sorts of contacts would I like to make?

Once you answer these questions, you can do a bit of recon to set yourself up for success before you arrive. Check out the conference website for listings of who else will be there. Conference organizers often provide professional biographies or websites and contact information for keynote speakers, presenters, and vendors. If you do some basic intel gathering—or even take it a step further and reach out to someone you'd like to meet ahead of time to lay the groundwork for a relationship—you'll arrive and meet that person prepared and can connect more genuinely. Guess how many people do this? Almost nobody. That means that if you do this, your person of interest will remember you. Ah, you clever master, you!

Fuel for Success

Have you ever tried to focus on studying or performing at the top of your game while starving? It wasn't very effective, was it? Packing simple snacks will prevent your growling stomach from hijacking your attention at an event. As a bonus, it will also likely save you unwanted calories or overpriced conference food. Here are some favorite recommendations that I've field tested and approved over the years:

- Jerky
- Protein bars
- Homemade yogurt parfaits
- Water (hydration is key!)
- Oatmeal (lifesaver!)

- Protein shakes (powder or ready-to-drink)
- Prepped meals (if so compelled)
- Trail mix
- Dried fruit
- Yogurt cups (Greek packs more protein)
- PB&J sandwich
- Money for eating out just in case (always come prepared!)

Sharp Body, Sharp Mind

I think you guys know me a little bit by now—how can we not talk about fitness? Keeping on your fitness game while at the conference doesn't have to be all Arnold Schwarzenegger style—keep it simple and on track. The brain works so much better with oxygen and movement. It can literally stimulate your best ideas and intellectual performance, case-in-point: the idea for writing this book! Some key items to pack for workouts at hotels include workout clothes/shoes, headphones, and a water bottle.

These are just a few simple solutions you can use so that you feel prepared when going into a conference. Now that the prep work has been addressed, let's dive into the best tips for nurturing your interactions *at* the conference!

PART II: CRUSH IT AT THE CONFERENCE

Okay, you have done all your prep work, you feel prepared, you have your targets set, and you are ready to go! Now it's time to put all of that prep into action. What you do and how you present yourself both verbally and nonverbally will dictate how people view you and your mission—your brand. You can make social media posts, script illustrious emails, and edit Oscar-worthy videos online, but how you show up *in person* lets people know the real, raw you. Your actions answer the question who is this person? That may sound like a lot of pressure, but it's reality, and recognizing this reality will set you far above those wandering around without a game plan.

Conference Day Checklist
Right before Heading to the Event

- ❏ Check yourself before you wreck yourself. Straighten your tie and give yourself a once-over. A big white string on the back of your black suit won't get you the kind of attention you want.
- ❏ Deodorant. This should be obvious, but sadly, it ain't.
- ❏ Perfume/cologne. It's always recommended to abstain so you don't offend your target, but I say you can show up with some swag. Just keep it subtle! One or two spritz, MAX. Don't go overboard or your contact may wish they could jump overboard!
- ❏ Keep your résumé/CV crisp and unwrinkled in a professional folder.
- ❏ Wear a nametag and consider professional, creative business cards.
- ❏ Carry at least two pens—one for you and one to make you look like a rock star if your target needs one. Trust me, I'm writing this in here for good reason!
- ❏ A copy of the event itinerary.
- ❏ Room key (don't lock yourself out!).
- ❏ Snacks, water bottle, magical coffee (this will save you from the lines and some money—almost every hotel has free coffee and a coffeemaker in your room).
- ❏ Get a fresh haircut a few days before the conference.

Ground Zero: The Eagle Has Landed
Conquer Your Confidence with Poise, Posture, and Presence

Whether you like it or not, the moment you step into a room, people immediately begin forming some sort of opinion about you. We are all wired to make snap judgments about others as fast as possible. It's a survival instinct we adopted long ago. What impression will you make? Are you genuine, a slob, out of place, professional? Almost all of these judgements are based on *how you carry yourself*.

If you enter the room with confidence and ease, people will be more inclined to give you attention and respect. But, if you roll in looking like you just rolled out of bed, you'll likely be instantly—if not irrevocably—discredited or written off by your peers.

It's the reality of social psychology. So, it's best to arrive equipped to take notes and play the game. That way you can become the master of your domain. It's not just about what clothes you wear, but also the *facial expression* and *posture* you display to the room. Repeat: do not ignore this. The way you carry yourself communicates everything!

According to research by Albert Mehrabian, non-verbal cues represent fifty-five percent of our communication. Vocal inflection is just thirty-eight percent, while our words constitute a mere seven percent. Perhaps you've heard the saying *actions speak louder than words*, and how true that cliché is! The seemingly most minute and irrelevant physical cues—from where your hands lie when you're sitting to how you cross your legs—set a tone. You want that tone to ring bright with success, warmth, and vibes that say, *I am someone you want to meet!* This can be best achieved by carrying yourself with confidence. It sounds simple enough, right? But simple does not mean easy, as many of us struggle with self-doubt. Not only that, but there is also the limiting belief that if you aren't born with confidence, then you're up the creek without a paddle. But I have good news. Paddles can be made! Self-confidence is a skill, something you can learn to convey to others. You can start by making small changes to your physical movements.

The following is a checklist to immediately boost your confidence vibes courtesy of Jan Hargrave, a renowned body language expert:

❑ Square Your Shoulders

If you're slouched or crouched, it displays a lack of confidence and even a lack of sincerity. Stand up straight, open up your chest fully and push your shoulders back slightly. Unevenness of shoulders suggests indecisiveness in a person. Square your shoulders toward your speaking partner. If you are speaking to another, but your body is facing away, it can appear discourteous or uncomfortable. Squaring off your shoulders towards your partner communicates a sense of interest and confidence.

❑ Stop the Fidgeting

This is a dead giveaway that you feel uncomfortable. Have you ever watched a professional newscaster? They never touch their face, adjust their ties, pull at their clothing, or play with their jewelry. If you seem nervous or insecure while delivering interacting, you lose trust and ease.

❑ Steeple Your Hands

A simple hand gesture can make you appear more confident and secure. Many people are used to what is called the "fig leaf" gesture, in which one hand cups the other and rests over the groin area. But this hand gesture actually conveys insecurity and weakness. The hand steeple, in which the fingers come together to form a point, is a great alternative. When someone steeples in the chest area, it means they are confident about what they are saying. When someone steeples in the lap area, it means they are confident about what they are hearing.

❑ Make Eye Contact

If you are having a one-on-one conversation, direct eye contact is critical. Follow the 80/20 rule, in which eighty percent of the time your eyes are meeting your speaking partner's and twenty percent of the time your eyes can roam as you gather information. Good eye contact allows your speaking partner to feel that you are interested in what they are saying. They will appreciate and respect you more and associate you as a caring, confident individual.

❑ Firm Your Handshake

A good handshake can set the tone for your following interaction with another individual. The best handshake starts with you holding your hand in a vertical position, with your fingers together and your thumb extended upright. Then, when shake your partner's hand, it must be a close, assertive connection in which the web of your hand meets his web. Be sure you approach their hand as evenly as possible. When someone's hand is facing down, it means they want to control you. And if their hand is facing up, it conveys that they are submissive. If you want to go the extra mile to convey confidence, try anchoring the handshake. This means using your other hand to touch the person softly on their forearm between their wrist and their elbow. Done correctly, this move can give an impression that you are fully committed to speaking with the person. Just be sure to not go any higher than the elbow, as this could make the person feel like you are invading their personal space.

A final word on communication...

Keep your eyes off your phone! Make each interaction about *them*, not you. *Those who are interested in others are the most interesting.* You are amazing and you have a lot to offer! And guess what? Everyone else thinks the same thing about themselves, and they want to connect as well. So, if you indulge them with your interest, guess who they'll remember? The person who rambled on about their sorority highlights and Rho Chi status, or the person who really listened and made them feel special? Remember the wise words of Maya Angelou, who stated that while people may forget what you said, they will never forget how you made them *feel*.

Ask *them* for their business card. This now positions the follow up as firmly within your control—*you* are now responsible for keeping the connection going, rather than relying on another person who has dozens of other business cards floating around in their pocket.

Business card hack

Get a business card from *them*! You can make an impression with your card but don't settle for simply giving business cards. How many dozens of other people do you think gave them their card too—especially if you're attending a networking event? When you give someone a business card, you are inherently saying *the follow up is in your hands and at your discretion.* I prefer a different approach.

> **Pro Tip:** If you want to follow up with someone, write a few key things that stuck out about the person you just met on the back of their card. Do this ASAP, like *now*—you want the details to be fresh. Since you'll likely be meeting a lot of people, there's a risk that the specifics for each individual will get lost or blurred together.

PART III: FOCUS ON THE FOLLOW-UP

You've done the prep work, you met interesting people, and you impressed them with your confidence and ability to listen. You have the tools and the stage is set. Now, you need to *act*! This is where ninety-nine percent of people drop the ball.

> But, Adam, the conference went great,
> I made some new contacts, now back to life as usual.

Now it's *game on!* You made the contact, you set the stage, you represented your personal brand well—now, *what are you going to do with it?*

Follow up email 101: The most basic course of action you should take after any event is to reach out to the contacts you made if you would like to foster relationships. Whether you are looking for a residency, potential job, or just a really interesting professional with whom you'd like to stay in contact, these are the most common must-keeps. Sending a thank-you email is a great gesture, and there are some keys to keep in mind before you hit the send button.

- **Grammar**: Nothing reads more unprofessional and lazy than sendin en email n'at wit turrible gramerrrrr that lukz like a text 2 ur friend. Who woud ever take you seriously!

- **Keep it professional**: Avoid first names, especially during this first reconnection. Using first names can come off as classless, and you are a classy professional! Stick with "Dr. Smith" or "Mrs. Smith." If you're not sure how to properly address them, check their business card, as they created it and it literally says how they prefer to be addressed. Turns out those business cards aren't just business cards at all, but cheat sheets for follow up!

- **Make it personal**: Focus on one specific feature that you genuinely appreciated about the interaction that will help your new contact remember you. For example, "I love that we both share a passion for fitness. It was great to learn about the recent marathon you ran last spring." This will serve two purposes. It will help them remember you and your face, and show them you were present in the conversation and listening to what they had to say. Remember, whoever is most interested becomes the most interesting. Reinforce why you stand out among the crowd. You are most welcome, you network ninja, you!

- **Think outside the inbox**: If you made a super special connection, or met someone from a key institution linked to a specific residency or job you are after, take your follow up to the next level by *sending a hand-written thank you card*. Yes, snail mail does still exist! Crazy, right? This will help you really stand out, because it inherently demonstrates just how much you care. If you take the extra effort to show your appreciation, whoever is on the other end will remember this interaction as a special one.

- **Connect on social media**: Learn LinkedIn! If you've been consistently building your personal brand, this is one of the times your hard work will really shine. When someone gets a request from you on social, and they glance over your account, what will they see? Funny cat videos or value-packed articles you wrote, podcast interviews, info memes, or blog recaps of conferences? Craft your brand and be so good they can't ignore you. It all matters.

EXERCISE:

Going to conferences is highly recommended, especially for pharmacy students trying to build their careers. If you've never been to one before, I recommend committing to go to at least one this year—the year you are reading this book! Pick one pharmacy organization with a platform in which you are interested and look at their upcoming conferences (*e.g., I resonate with SNPhA, which has a platform that serves the underserved. They have one regional and one national meeting per year, and right now as a P2, I can commit to the regional meeting. I went to their website and registered*).

The one pharmacy organization that I most resonate with is:

_____

_____

_____

_____

_____

_____

_____

I looked at their website and conference options this year are:

_____

_____

_____

_____

_____

_____

_____

_____

I am committed to creating a network to grow and expand my career. And, because nothing grows in the comfort zone, I have committed to register to attend this conference—and I cannot wait!

Chapter 10

THE THREE LEVELS OF MENTORSHIP

*"Formal education will make you a living;
self-education will make you a fortune."*

—Jim Rohn

I LOVE WHERE I went to school! Not because of the sports teams or the parties, but because of the quality of education and superb support system the school offers their students.

There are many good pharmacy schools across the United States, but for me, the University of Pittsburgh School of Pharmacy is unmatched in the complete quality of education. The curriculum is well-organized, diverse, and enhanced by the caring solid support system of both faculty and students. Their goal is clear: equip you to learn, succeed, and grow as a leader in the pharmacy profession.

I could write a book about why the school is so unique in helping students succeed in developing leadership qualities that business owners and corporations dream about when hiring, but even *that* would not do the school justice. However, I believe the key to successful development is not just the school's responsibility. You have to be resourceful in leveraging your experience wherever you attend pharmacy school.

> But, Adam, I don't get along with my professors.
> The people in my class just aren't my type.
> No one in my school really gets me or my vision.

These realities may seem like they'll inevitably lead to a downtrodden mental funk, but fear not! If the environment you are in now is not fully supportive or nurturing of your vision or goals, I have phenomenal news. You can create your own new environment crafted exactly how you want it to look and feel! Support, guidance, inspiration—how do those feelings sound? If your current environment is lacking these uplifting qualities, I invite you to look at the bigger picture.

You can open up endless possibilities for resources, connection, and network building with students outside of your profession and even from other pharmacy schools. Better yet, be the change you want to see in your program! Meet with faculty, talk with fellow students, and create a movement. Be a leader!

When you love and connect to your school, faculty, program, and peers, you have the opportunity to cultivate mentoring relationships. I mentioned that I became involved in the Student National Pharmaceutical Association (SNPhA). Its parent organization for pharmacists is the National Pharmaceutical Organization (NPhA), and their slogan states the following:

"SNPhA is dedicated to the pharmacy profession and serving the underserved."

One reason I love Pitt Pharmacy so much is that I owe this organization a ton of credit for the amazing opportunities it afforded me, not only a pharmacy student, but also as a pre-pharmacy student where my journey began, and now pharmacist where my journey continues.

I had the honor to host a workshop in Houston, Texas, at the 2019 SNPhA Annual Convention, guiding pharmacy students through my speaking program on the three levels of mentorship topic of this very chapter. It was standing room only, and while the program was only an hour long, pharmacy students stayed for almost two hours afterward to connect, ask questions, and create momentum for their personal brand.

That is what I find so exceptional about this organization—you can become involved at every level of your education. If you do not have a SNPhA chapter at your pharmacy school, guess who could start one?

You can shift your entire environment and it all starts with one email, direct message, or phone call. Take action and express your interest. You may have to search, you may have to build, or you may be already surrounded by incredible mentors, but you *do* have to engage.

Let's say you have successfully found your tribe and you are involved in an organization with a mission and values that speak to you. I suggest looking for one-on-one mentorship. The answer to finding a mentor may be as simple as looking up from your notes in class (*wake up, you—shhh, I won't tell*).

Mentorship doesn't have to be a formal process. Build a relationship with your professor or colleague you respect. Show up. Hang around. Ask for help. *Get involved* with what they're doing.

If this seems too daunting, or unlikely to work for your circumstances, I've got you covered, FitPharmFam. The entire second half of this book is a collection of interviews for you, conducted *by* pharmacy students. The interviews highlight amazing pharmacy heavyweights who will inspire you and guide you with decades of experience and expertise. Imagine getting to know professionals like this personally. *That* is mentorship!

Mentorship is something I would define as *priceless* to someone pursuing a career. A mentor provides guidance, confidence, and a two-way learning relationship. Yes, the teacher does become the student! The teacher once took the path that the student is now taking—they experienced many of the same difficulties, setbacks, joys and epiphanies along the way—and they're just waiting to share with you.

Finding a mentor can feel awkward or uneasy, so let me share how I found my first mentor in pharmacy.

I have enjoyed organizing and planning projects and events ever since I became an Eagle Scout at the age of fourteen. Once I decided I wanted to become a pharmacist, I joined a pharmacy organization that paired pre-pharmacy students with students enrolled in the school of pharmacy to offer mentorship. One goal was to assist undergraduates in meeting admittance requirements for pharmacy school.

While attending these meetings, I noticed how good the president was at conducting meetings, delivering information, and communicating with co-chairs. I took a risk and introduced myself. I was a total stranger who stepped up to shake hands, introduce myself, and ask for help. That got his attention. Lucky for me, he took me under his wing, and he soon became my mentor and good friend, still to this day. Did I formally ask him to be my mentor? No. Our relationship grew and he filled that role and need in my life.

I met my second mentor as a student in pharmacy school. When I realized that I really loved teaching, I approached my favorite professor. From all the questions and conversation throughout subsequent years, we formed a relationship whereby she shared all of her wisdom and experience with me. She helped demonstrate how I could best develop my own teaching abilities. We are still friends to this day, and she has been the guiding voice that enabled the initial framework for the book idea you now hold in your hands.

I share these stories to offer three pieces of advice:

1. **Take the initiative**—don't just go through the motions and follow the syllabus. Yes, grades are important, but so is what you do *outside* of the classroom.

2. **Don't let fear limit you**—nothing good is ever easy, and there are no free lunches (except for the samples at Costco). So step up for yourself. The only thing holding you back is you—take that leap and reap the rewards!

3. **Do it now**—if you don't connect with potential mentors, you may miss life-changing advice, support, and opportunities.

If you have reached a point in your career where you believe you have something valuable that could help other students learn, I beg you to please give back. It is a privilege to act as a mentor just like it is a privilege to be mentored. Return the favor to future generations!

Make a difference in someone's life. Lead by example. Others will follow your footsteps, not your words. Leave a legacy of one lasting relationship at a time. Even as a student, someone desperately needs your help.

EXERCISE:

What area of pharmacy do you find most interesting?

_____

_____

_____

_____

_____

What professor or upperclassman in your school do you know who specializes in this area of study?

_____

_____

_____

_____

_____

Set up a brief meeting to introduce yourself via email or direct message, or if they are a current professor, walk up after class and introduce yourself and express your interest in their field. Ask for a meeting to speak more about career path options!

I connected with the professor, and we are scheduled to meet on _____ **.**

Chapter 11

....

LEADERSHIP & LEGACY

*"To handle yourself, use your head;
to handle others, use your heart."*

—Eleanor Roosevelt

AS PHARMACISTS, we integrate skill sets ranging from counseling, finance, business, communication, psychology, pharmacology, engineering—the list goes on and on! One skill ties all the others together. That one skill, if mastered, can enhance any other skill you hope to improve. That skill is *leadership*.

Pharmacists are a part of a team. Your team works together in all that you do to deliver the best care possible to your patients, accurately fill prescriptions, minimize medication safety errors, and cut unnecessary costs. To do all this, you need to effectively lead your team of technicians, pharmacists, interns, and support personnel. No one can do everything—*each needs the help of the other!*

Effectively managing people is the greatest challenge you may ever face professionally. Empowering and aligning each team member with their inherent strengths and preferences is easier said than done. Doing that will best set you up for long-term success. Focusing on trust, respect, and effectiveness with everyone on your team is the core of how to do this. There will be new tasks and challenges every day, but it is your team—together—that must cohesively and happily create a long-term winning environment.

Leadership isn't just being nice, it is a *science*. There is theory, practice, and even research to back that up. By looking at research and studies published by experts in the field, I present to you a way to warm your leadership skills and get social with your team: the SCARF model.

Let's get basic for a minute and return to elementary school. Do you remember back in recess when you were left out of a sports game, sleepover, or secret club meeting in the treehouse? It felt pretty crappy, right? You may have even cried. I did! As it turns out, *the feeling of being excluded elicits the same reaction in the brain as physical pain!*

This link between physical and social pain is tied to one of our three basic psychological needs: relatedness. Researcher Matthew Lieberman hypothesizes this is the case because "...being socially connected to caregivers is necessary for survival." Social interaction is hardwired as a *need* in our brains.

How can we apply this to pharmacy school and your future workplace as a pharmacist to become an effective leader? Keeping your pharmacy team engaged and feeling socially in-tune with each other can play a huge role in your team's performance. If a team member is in social pain, this will limit their commitment to the initiatives and the roles required to deliver high performance.

How can a leader prevent social pain from happening? Knowing each colleague on a personal level plays a huge role, because you want to strive to align each individual's talents with tasks that must be completed. On an even more personal level from their perspective, it's being appreciated. We all want to feel known and needed. Returning to the pharmacy team environment, we want to avoid mismatching talents and tasks, but we also want to lead a cohesive team that works together because they're happy and like each other. That is how we can deliver the best patient care and fulfill our roles as one unit.

> But, Adam, my techs bicker! She will never come around!
> He just doesn't get along with anyone!

If these are your first reactions when thinking about your work environment, a *threat response* has likely been triggered. Understanding how to manage that is what we will dive into next.

EXERCISE

Reflect on a time in your life when you felt isolated as an outsider of a group. How did that make you feel? Were you giving your best self to the group and helping to achieve the goal of the team at your full capacity? Why or why not?

_____

_____

_____

_____

_____

_____

_____

Reflect on a time in the last year where there was disconnect among a team with which you were involved. Describe the scenario and dynamics below.

_____

_____

_____

_____

_____

_____

_____

After reading your scenario, could it have been that the antagonist in your scenario (the trouble-maker) felt isolated or threatened in some way? If you were to have focused on addressing that need first, what would the dynamic likely have been instead?

_____

_____

_____

_____

_____

_____

_____

Chapter 12

BUILD YOUR TEAM AS A PHARMACY LEADER

"A leader is one who knows the way, goes the way, and shows the way."

—John C. Maxwell

THIS CHAPTER ties in with your group work as a pharmacy student, your role as a leader on your clinical rotations, and as a future pharmacist leading your team. If you practice the following now as a student, and use your time in pharmacy school to implement them in your professional group work, it will soon become second-nature over time and will pay major dividends to your leadership development.

If a group member on a team feels threatened, they will not function at optimal productivity. The key to being an effective leader is ensuring the opposite of the threat response occurs. How can we do that? We *enable the reward response*. Each team member must feel important and rewarded for their presence, effort, and input. Focus on five qualities that empower the reward response and shut off the threat response: **SCARF!**

Status
Certainty
Autonomy
Relatedness
Fairness

Status

Anyone hooked on the Kardashians is not likely raving about their extreme intelligence—it's their social status that is so alluring. How does status translate in the pharmacy setting? If a coworker feels like they are of lower status to someone else, this ignites a threat response. On the flipside, the belief you are highly regarded by your peers leads to feelings of reward. Believe it or not, a feeling of high status actually correlates with longevity and health, as described in Michael Marmot's book *The Status Syndrome: How Social Standing Affects Our Health and Longevity.*

How do you approach your team when giving feedback? One big trigger is saying, *let me show you how to do it the right way.* This statement is almost always interpreted as a threat, because its underlying implication is *I am superior, and you are doing it all wrong.* Perhaps you have heard the adage, sandwich your critiques in praise? This is why that advice is so effective! Giving people praise strengthens their perception of high status, making them more receptive to the constructive criticism you may be offering. We are only trying to help our team become better, but approaching this goal the wrong way can create a toxic work environment and literally cause pain. Approach with praise and watch your team grow!

Certainty

We don't always know how a day will pan out—often our grand plan never comes close to materializing the way we pictured it in our mind. However, having some level of certainty can put our minds at ease and allow us to put energy into being productive instead of worrying. This rings so true in the world of pharmacy. We should strive to set clear expectations with our team right up front for the scenario of organized chaos we all know a pharmacy can be. The key word there is organized. Who is going to type in prescriptions? Who will be in charge of ringing up patients for their order at the register? Who is going to be in charge of inventory management? What's for lunch? What is a lunch break, anyway?

Setting and clearly communicating these roles to your team will ease tension by fostering a basic workplace certainty.

Autonomy

We have all had one of those bosses who takes the whole creating certainty a bit too far for our liking. Maybe they wanted to dictate how many breaths you should take per minute or what you should do in your free time. Think back to that experience—how did it make you feel? Frustrated, angry, maybe even excessively controlled? Your feeling of autonomy was threatened. Overreaching or micro-managing employees can cause an unbearably stressful environment. But it does not have to be that way!

Yes, guidance and direction are paramount to success, but allowing your team to feel they can complete assigned tasks using their *own* decisions and judgement without someone looking over their shoulder provides a sense of empowerment. It's not that you need to let everyone run wild, but the key is that people *feel* they have autonomy. There is a line between providing certainty and allowing autonomy. Maintaining an open network of communication will prevent this balance from tilting and becoming problematic.

Relatedness

Feeling like you belong to a team will make you more inclined to want to work to make that team perform at a higher level. If you don't feel like you're a needed member, what incentive do you have to want to improve the group? This simple concept has profound implications for work and colleague engagement in ClubPharmacy! If someone feels like they are a part of a group, they will have more trust and empathy for initiatives set when working toward a goal.

> But, Adam, everyone is so different!
> How can I expect them all to get along?

The ease at which teamwork occurs can vary greatly from group to group. Two helpful ingredients that can overcome distance or bad feelings between colleagues are time and repeated social interaction. This feeling of comfort is related to the amount of oxytocin released by the brain in the presence of people with whom we are most comfortable. A release of oxytocin diffuses the threat response and allows bonding and accepting others as a part of our group. Research using exogenous dosing of oxytocin has demonstrated the impact this feeling has on our interactions with other people by minimizing the threat response.

As pharmacy leaders, if we work to eliminate feelings of isolation and ensure everyone feels included as equal members of a team, we can foster an ideal environment that augments productivity and team effort.

Fairness

If one pharmacy technician is ten minutes late and you say nothing, but another tech is ten minutes late and they get scolded, how do you think the scolded tech will feel? How do you think other techs will perceive that environment? This perceived unfairness could evoke feelings of threat or uncertainty, which we now know thwarts productivity.

This impact has been represented through studies conducted by Lieberman and Tabibnia. They found that people respond more favorably when given $0.50 from a $1 split between them and one other person, even when compared to receiving $8 out of $25 between two people. Wait, what?

In the second scenario, where people were shown $25 and given $8, they were given significantly more money compared to the group who received only $0.50 of the $1 initially shown. So why the angst? Even though it was more money, *it was not perceived as fair*, and that is our human default. Apply the findings of this to your work in pharmacy school organizations and ClubPharmacy dynamics and you may see the impact that perceived fairness can have on your team's cohesiveness.

One way to ensure an environment of fairness and equality among your team is through *transparency*. Communicate your plans, actions, and intentions to keep everyone on the same page. Even when times get tough (this is the pharmacy world, after all), a well-established environment of transparency will mean the lows aren't as low as they would be had this comradery not been developed and engrained in your pharmacy culture.

Does the SCARF fit? One size fits all?

Being a pharmacist is a tremendous responsibility and it requires you step into the role of leadership. Each and every action you take will be analyzed by your team, and you will, in essence, lead by example. That can feel either overwhelming or empowering. You have the power to make profound impacts on your pharmacy by improving teamwork and delivering the best patient care possible through working together as one unit.

Threat and reward responses are real—the threat response is strong, urgent, and cannot be ignored. Mitigating the stress response and shifting power to the reward response resides in following the concepts of the SCARF model.

You don't have to wait until you're a pharmacist to build a team—in fact, it's optimal to start now as a student. Group projects, study groups, and other team work opportunities will be available throughout pharmacy school. Remind yourself about the mentorship process and implement what you have learned in this chapter—you literally will be building a support team...just...like...when you're a pharmacist and you are building and leading a team.

By following this model, you will become a more effective leader and a better pharmacist capable of your ultimate task to provide the best level of care possible to your patients. Your future patients are worth it!

EXERCISE

Looking at the SCARF model we just discussed, reflect on your interactions you have with your peers in pharmacy school. With the five components in mind, which one do you feel needs more attention in your interactions as a pharmacy student? If you make this a focal point to improve, how will this impact your ability to serve as a leader?

_____

_____

_____

_____

_____

_____

Now let's apply the SCARF model to where you work as an intern. Do you see the same component(s) lacking implementation in this environment, or is there a different one that needs addressed? If you took ownership to improve this dynamic, how do you think it would impact your work environment and ability to serve as a leader?

_____

_____

_____

_____

Chapter 13

DISPENSE YOUR FULL POTENTIAL AS A LEADER

"The only person you can control is you. So focus on making yourself who you want to be: Faster. Smarter. Stronger. More humble. Less ego."

—Jocko Willink

TO LEARN HOW to lead most effectively, why not delve into the most extreme environment, where every command can literally translate to life or death: Navy SEAL team leaders in the Iraq war. A book I highly recommend is *Extreme Ownership: How U.S. Navy SEALs Lead and Win* by authors Jocko Willink and Leif Babin. They share their experiences of leadership through life-threatening environments and break down the concepts they used when leading their teams. You can apply them to raising a family, running a pharmacy team, or just about every part of life!

℞ 1: Take Extreme Ownership of *Everything* in Your Life

To be an effective leader, you must first admit your failures and refrain from blaming others. Set aside your excuses and reflect honestly. Regroup. Evaluate. But accept responsibility. Taking full responsibility for both your actions *and* the actions of those you lead requires humility and courage—qualities that will make you an effective leader beyond measure. Simply, if it's important to you, you'll find a way—if not, you'll find an excuse.

℞ 2: Lead by Example

There are no bad teams—only bad leaders. As a leader, you are in charge, and people will follow your lead. The standards you set for yourself and others are all up to you. Live them. One goal you should set, one that is the true test of good leadership, is training your team so well that they function without needing you to be there. If you step away from the helm, will your team persist or crumble without your guidance?

℞ 3: Your Why Must Be Clearly Understood and Communicated

As we learned at the very beginning of this book, the why should be the driving force behind every action—especially when you encounter an obstacle or difficulty. Focus on the *why* instead of a person and watch your team follow through with the objective.

℞ 4: Check Yourself Before You Wreck Yourself

There is a clear difference between confidence and arrogance. The main distinction has to do with your ego. Stay humble! Confidence rooted in humility attracts loyalty and teamwork. Arrogance undermines it.

℞ 5: The Secret to Success is Simplicity

Overcomplicating anything leads to confusion, poor communication, and more problems than solutions. *Clarity creates power*, so ensure every member of your team understands the mission and the why. Continually work to simplify the objective.

6: Trust Your Team through Actions of Delegation

There is only so much you can do to influence people directly. One person can only effectively manage six to ten people according to research by David Rock. That may sound limiting, but you can, and should, *delegate*. Those to whom you delegate responsibilities need to understand the limits of their authority as well.

7: Proper Planning Prevents Poor Performance

The first thing when approaching a mission is to analyze your objective—remember your *why*. Here it is again! Lay out your plan of attack, be methodical, expect setbacks, delegate, take action, and then assess outcomes. Be S.M.A.R.T. about your goals!

S.M.A.R.T. goals
Specific
Measurable
Achievable
Realistic
Time-bound

8: Do Not Allow Uncertainty to Stall Your Actions

Rarely will you be one hundred percent certain of every decision you make as a leader. Rather than not taking action due to analysis paralysis, instead make the best decision you can with the intel you have. If you wait for the perfect situation to act, you will never act. The time to act is now!

9: Discipline Will Keep You Moving Forward

Leading requires embodying numerous dichotomies: "...aggressive but not overbearing; quiet but not silent; calm but not robotic; humble but not passive; competitive but a gracious loser." Maintain awareness of yourself and others through emotional intelligence and leadership experience will empower you to find the balance that's right for you.

10: Constant and Never-Ending Improvement

This final concept comes straight from me, FitPharmFam. If you read my book R_x: *YOU! The Pharmacist's Survival Guide for Managing Stress & Fitting in Fitness*, you have heard this concept before. Quite simply, if you're not growing, you're dying. As a leader, one of your core responsibilities is to lead your team to growth. If *you* are not growing, how can you expect to lead others to grow? Commit to getting one percent better every single day. The key is not how much you can grow in one day, but how *consistent* you make personal development over time. As Matthew Kelly once said, most people overestimate what they can do in a day, and underestimate what they can do in a month. We overestimate what we can do in a year, and underestimate what we can accomplish in a decade.

You cannot take care of others if you don't first take care of yourself. You cannot pour from an empty cup.

Don't try to figure out whether the cup is half empty or half full—figure out how you can make the cup overflow with abundance so that you can give to an even greater degree to those whom you serve.

EXERCISE

Looking at the ten principles you just read, which do you feel that you excel at implementing as a leader?

_____

_____

_____

_____

_____

_____

Now, take an honest assessment of your qualities as a leader. Which of the ten principles discussed in this chapter do you feel need to be improved in your life?

_____

_____

_____

_____

_____

_____

_____

_____

Chapter 14

THE LONG GAME

"The seed of a bamboo tree is planted, fertilized, and watered. Nothing happens for the first year. There´s no sign of growth. Not even a hint. The same thing happens—or doesn´t happen—the second year. And then the third year. The tree is carefully watered and fertilized each year, but nothing shows. No growth. No anything. For eight years it can continue. Eight years! Then—after the eight years of fertilizing and watering have passed, with nothing to show for it—the bamboo tree suddenly sprouts and grows thirty feet in three months!"

—Zig Ziglar

I'M TRYING to focus on three things in my healthcare career. I want them to ground me. I want them to be my anchors in the storms of my life. I want them to be my legacy.

I hope they will empower *you* to live at *your* highest potential. Maybe we can look at them as a personal standard of practice. A shared agreement. In my pharmacy career, I first began working as a technician, then pharmacy intern, and now I serve as a pharmacist. Throughout my journey, I have had the privilege to both observe and learn from a wide array of professionals in all stages of their careers. I noticed two polar opposites when it came to their outcomes: either burnout or resentment for the profession leading to a bitter career change, or a feeling of true fulfilled purpose—that feeling of *I was born to do this*.

Regardless of the outcome, I noticed what things led to the former so as to avoid them, and to a greater point of focus, what habits led to the latter. In fact, my curiosity for what makes the best of the best in pharmacy stand out led to the creation of *The Fit Pharmacist Healthcare Podcast*. Available on all podcast platforms, this weekly podcast functions to bring the best tips to practice pharmacy and create a fulfilling career through inspiring interviews with the highest-performing professionals in healthcare. This passion to learn how to live a fulfilled pharmacy career—and share that knowledge with our profession—led me to be named the Most Influential Pharmacist by SingleCare®'s Best of the Best Pharmacy Awards in 2019. *You* can have impact when you make it your mission and raise your standard to focus on learning how to dispense your full potential. The specific standards I have come to learn and adopt into my own practice deserve their own chapter, and that's what we are going to dive into now.

1. I Strive to be Impeccable with My Word

Words have the power to create, and they also have the power to destroy.

Let's agree to conduct ourselves with the realization that our words have power and other people's words have power.

Let's speak in a way that we can respect when the words come from our mouths when communicating with others and ourselves.

You've heard the saying *you are the sum of the five people with whom you spend the most time.* I want to speak about people not present in a way I would speak in their presence. I want to consume and speak words that empower us, not harm.

2. I Strive to Assess Emotions and Intentions

When we take things personally, we often feel offended and then react by defending. Conflict ensues. An argument, a war, hurt feelings, a broken relationship—always conflict.

The sad part is that despite countless belief systems and world views, endless personality combinations, completely unique life experiences, and sometimes unspeakable hurt, most of us share the exact same values. If we seek to *understand first*, and to be understood with reciprocal compassion, harmony rules. What better first impulse for a healthcare provider?

I want to assess my emotions before I speak or react. I want to understand the intent of others and our shared values. I want to create harmony not division.

3. I Strive to Dispense My Full Potential

How I speak to others is a mirror—a reflection of my attitude and a measurement of selflessness and service.

How I act is a direct response of either self-promotion and insecurity or empathy and care.

How I think is creating my existence moment by moment. How I think today is who I will be tomorrow. I want to be exceptional. I want to be exceptional, as I will be empowered to dispense my full potential to my patients, my family, my friends, to you, and to me.

How about it? Do we have a deal—an agreement? Let's strive to thrive.

> *"There are three masteries that lead people to become Toltecs. First is the Mastery of Awareness. This is to be aware of who we really are, with all the possibilities.*
>
> *The second is the Mastery of Transformation—how to change, how to be free of domestication.*
>
> *The third is the Mastery of Intent. Intent from the Toltec*

point of view is that part of life that makes transformation of energy possible; it is the one living being that seamlessly encompasses all energy, or what we call 'God.'
Intent is life itself; it is unconditional love.
The Mastery of Intent is therefore
the Mastery of Love."

—Miguel Ruiz

If you feel you gravitate toward negativity, self-limiting beliefs, or a lack of confidence, here is your R_x for awareness:

"Develop awareness of all the self-limiting, fear-based beliefs that make you unhappy. You take an inventory of all that you believe, all your agreements, and through this process you begin the transformation."

—Miguel Ruiz

EXERCISE

Craft your personal mission statement.

I strive...

PART II

Script Your Career—Experts Speak

PART II

....

22 FORMULAS FOR A FULFILLING CAREER

"If I have seen further than others, it is by standing upon the shoulders of giants."

—Sir Isaac Newton

A GUIDE WILL not only make life's journey less burdensome, but it will save you massive amounts of time in accomplishing your goals by following the footsteps of those who have already traveled the journey you are looking to begin. Yes, everyone lives a different path and purpose, but if you can glean just one golden nugget of knowledge from someone who is performing the skill you are looking to master, isn't that alone worth it? You do not have to reinvent the wheel, just trailblaze a path toward your inner greatness.

While this list is not all-inclusive, or meant to replace in-person or one-on-one mentorship, I hope it serves to open your mind to the vast possibilities for your pharmacy career. It is powerful advice from some of the most successful minds within their respective niche. I challenge you to not focus only on your specialty of interest, but to give each a chance by reading and learning from some of the best experts in our profession. Some may just surprise you in a good and unexpected way. It may shatter a previous thought and open your mind to a place of curiosity. I invite you to dive deeper into the endless opportunity this amazing profession holds for your career as a pharmacist, however you choose to be most fulfilled in serving your patients, community, and the world.

The following chapters are collections of interviews from some of the most popular areas in the profession of pharmacy. These interviews were graciously conducted by pharmacy students at the University of Pittsburgh School of Pharmacy, affording them the opportunity to have the experience of speaking with these brilliant minds in their own quest of improvement. Many thanks to Dean Dr. Patricia Kroboth for this brilliant idea to assign pharmacy students to perform the interviews as a way to enrich their experience in learning from their talented colleagues.

Happy exploring—the world (and profession) is your oyster, my friend!

SPECIALTY PHARMACY

Joshua S. Stoneking, PharmD
Regional Director, Oncology/Hematology (East/Gulf Coast)

Josh is an award-winning pharmacist for a growing Inc. 5000 specialty Pharmacy, who uses his unique knowledge to create partnerships in his respective territories. Josh is passionate about the needs and goals of his partnering clinics, specializing in bringing a peace of mind and superlative value to clinics that have previously struggled using other specialty pharmacy services. He takes pride in building a team atmosphere and always goes the extra mile to provide his patients with the highest level of specialty care. By making an industry leap from a clinical pharmacist to a specialty pharmacy director, Josh found professional success at a high level, earning his company's highest awards in oncology three years in a row.

Currently, he coaches and leads a strong team of exceptionally skilled regional account managers and operational experts across the east and gulf coasts. Josh earned his Bachelor of Science degree in Exercise Physiology and his Doctorate of Pharmacy degree from West Virginia University School of Medicine while completing his PGY-1 residency training at Indian River Medical Center in Vero Beach, Florida. He resides in the Washington D.C. metro area but maintains his original West "by God" Virginia roots.

In your own words, what exactly is "specialty pharmacy" as a niche profession?

Specialty pharmacy is a type of pharmacy that handles mainly specialty drugs. In this, the main disease states that specialty covers include, but are not limited to, oncology, infectious disease (HIV, hepatitis C), fertility, growth hormone, inflammation, some transplant medications, and pain management.

Also, specialty pharmacy involves compounding, as we can

compound ophthalmology drugs, and for government law 503B, we can compound bulk medications to give to a hospital for sale, although it's not patient-specific. With this practice, we must stay current with the USP 797 guidelines, and in my facility we have seventy-eight hoods to compound medications.

With the medications we deal with, we have highly-toxic, highly-priced, limited-access drugs. You won't find your common community pharmacy prescription orders for Percocet® or hydrochlorothiazide here.

When you compare the standard retail pharmacy versus specialty pharmacy clinic, it provides services to the clinic free of charge. The pharmacy can legally do prior authorizations for the clinic, in addition to seeking financial assistance for the patient. As the specialty medications are significantly more expensive than those commonly found in the retail setting, we as a specialty pharmacy can seek funding on the patient's behalf by going through government grants or private foundations. Examples of these channels include the Patient Access Network (PAN) and Leukemia & Lymphoma Society (LLS), which are service-based resources, not contract-based.

Looking at the clinical services side of specialty, each medication can involve three to five clinical calls a month per patient, depending on the cycle of the medication (i.e., chemotherapy cycle) and specific guidelines and standards of practice. In some rare disease states, follow-up is four to six weeks later, not immediately.

Technology has really advanced the capabilities of service with specialty pharmacy. For example, there now are *smart bottles* that light up when a medication dose is due to be taken, and will send you a text when the dose is due. The exact date and time the medication taken is sent to pharmacy so that we can monitor compliance and adherence in case a pharmacist needs to check in prior to the scheduled follow-up to ensure optimal care and to address potential barriers to the prescribed medication regimen.

What is your role as a pharmacist in specialty?

I serve as a clinical pharmacist, which in specialty pharmacy is disease state specific, as my main role. Whatever disease state you are in, that is all you will touch due to the highly-involved intricacies of the medications that we dispense. In a sense, it is very similar to a retail pharmacist's role, but we also are calling to do prior authorizations, assist in writing letters of medical necessity, partner with clinics as a consultant pharmacist, and sometimes go and counsel patients at clinics. Clinical follow-up calls are also part of the job.

Along with my main role, I am also a business development pharmacist, whereby I seek pharmaceutical company contracts and payor contracts for the specialty pharmacy company. With this role, I have to stay ahead of the game to see what drugs are coming out—health economics. I also work as a pharmacist in sales, so I am considered to be an outside sales representative as a licensed pharmacist. With this, I have to grow a territory, which is very similar to a pharmaceutical representative.

Why do you enjoy contributing to the profession through this specialty? Tell us what gets you excited about your work!

Mostly it's the joy of the level of freedom I have in serving my patients. By having split roles, I am not only taking care of the patients and providing them with the newest groundbreaking therapies, but I get to fight the insurance companies to get patients a drug that initially would have cost them $5,000 for only $10. I get to truly monitor them as if I was in the clinic, and with that I get to build that patient-pharmacist relationship.

The outcomes that I get to witness first-hand in working with rare disease states is remarkable, as I can truly tell if the level of the patients' health has improved from my interventions.

From the business development role, I love the traveling, contracting with hospitals and cancer centers, and giving continuing education presentations. Every pharmacist in specialty pharmacy has multiple roles, and that is what I love about specialty pharmacy most.

What are the current requirements/certifications to practice in this specialty niche as a pharmacist?

You must have your PharmD degree or RPh, along with some sort of disease state-specific experience or training, and this depends on your specialty. For example, having a pain management certification, BCOP, or BCPS—it all is specific to your disease state area of expertise as a specialty pharmacist. None of this is required, but it will set you apart and serve you well. Or, once you are in a specialty company, you tend to get those trainings/certifications as well. Also, once your company contracts to provide a specialty medication, you will get training from the pharmaceutical companies who make that drug. So really, the only requirement is to be a registered pharmacist or have your PharmD.

In regards to a residency for specialty pharmacy, it is not required. Having disease state-specific certification/training will really help your career options, and compounding experience will probably be the most important.

If you could go back to your first day of pharmacy school, and knew that you would end up in specialty pharmacy, what steps would you take to build your professional résumé to best align you for success?

I would definitely have taken more business classes, and pursued the masters in business administration option. I wish I paid more attention to how insurance companies work with regards to the prior authorization process behind the scenes and what makes a prior authorization. Having more prior authorization and insurance knowledge would have lessened the learning curve for sure. I wish that earlier on in pharmacy school I knew more about specialty pharmacy, or that it even existed! I would have—and recommend that you—dive deeper into pharmacy as early on in your career as possible. It will be worth it!

What organizations, publications, or establishments would you recommend to follow to build a strong repertoire and/or better familiarize yourself with being an effective pharmacist in the specialty niche?

I would recommend the National Association of Specialty Pharmacy (NASP)—they hold a convention in Washington, D.C., every year. I highly recommend that you take action to get involved by going to it!

If you are looking into oncology, the National Comprehensive Cancer Network (NCCN) guidelines are your bible—get involved in all of oncology-specific branches. Overall, all organizations are disease state-specific, so you'll want to first identify which disease state you are looking to dive deeper into from the clinical side.

From the business side, you need to get in and build your own personal network. Learn about business development and insurance through your company that you work at as in intern; look for shadow opportunities and do whatever you can to immerse yourself and learn about how business works.

Are there any suggestions you would make to a first-year pharmacy student to better prepare them or give them a good overview, or glimpse, if you will, into the "real world" of specialty pharmacy?

Do your due diligence of what a specialty pharmacy is, as currently, due to the lack of information that is out there, it is not as prolific as community or hospital pharmacy information.

For a real-world view of specialty pharmacy, know that you are going to be filling less medications, but the filling process will be a lot longer (e.g., three to five business days), and you will often feel more like a lawyer than a pharmacist at times.

You will be building a lot of cases to insurance companies and the government (for grants) as well.

From the patient-care focus, you will not have as many patients walking through your door, as you will mostly mail prescription orders to your patients, as ninety percent of specialty drugs need to be shipped. You do not need to focus on retail skills to be in specialty—you need to focus on your clinical skills, so be sure to hone in on clinical excellence.

Also, make sure you take interest in the rare stuff! Prepare to be on the cutting edge of pharmacy!

What have you found to be the best strategy for performing "deep work"—that is, focused time spent to efficiently produce quality results to advance your career?

Simply, you must create a plan. This is a must, not an option. I find it most beneficial to make both a daily and weekly plan so that you can prioritize to get most important daily task done first, and be cautious not to let things carry over from your task list. It's not about having the time—you must always make time.

Don't just rush along to get things done—take pride in your work.

Show up with a positive attitude—this is an absolute must!

Challenge yourself to take on the new roles, and take the risk toward growth and learning new things. When there is change, accept the change. Volunteer for the new role that you are scared of, because if you fail, at least you will learn something new. Speaking of fear, do not be scared to be a leader. There is no *one right way* to lead—there are many ways to be an effective leader. You have to get started to gain experience, so put it out there! Let leadership know what your long-term, future goals are and be clear in your expectations through communication.

What overall suggestion would you make to become poised in the specialty niche of the profession of pharmacy throughout a student's time in pharmacy school?

Find the rare disease state that interests you most and find your desire to be on the forefront of treatment. Be ready to be fighting to get every new cure to the patients immediately and inexpensively as your duty and obligation.

Any final thoughts?

Being in pharmacy school is a fantastic opportunity—you may be frustrated or find times where you think pharmacy is not for you, but pharmacy is not just retail or clinic. There is a role out there for you!

This degree is so respected and sought after, no matter how many pitfalls you have, please stick it out and see it through, as your PharmD will give you the best option for a high-quality life. There will be a job for you—all you have to do is put in the work, stay consistent, and don't give up!

Many thanks to Dr. Joshua Stoneking for his time in sharing his expertise on his roles, responsibilities, and best-practice tips in the specialty niche of pharmacy, and for student pharmacist Maria Langas, who led this interview.

COMMUNITY PHARMACY I

Mike Corvino, PharmD, BCPS, CDE

Clinical Pharmacist at Franklin C. Fetter Family Health
Founder of CorConsult R$_x$

Dr. Corvino is a clinical pharmacist and certified diabetes educator for Fetter Health Care Network, as well as a diabetes educator for Palmetto Pharmacist Network. He serves as an adjunct pharmacology professor for the physician assistant program at Charleston Southern University. In 2017, he created CorConsultR$_x$ for the purpose of distributing evidence-based medicine updates and promoting continual education through various social media platforms. At the end of 2017, the CorConsultR$_x$ Flash Briefing was launched in the Alexa Skills Store through Amazon. This was followed by the CorConsultR$_x$ Podcast, which is now available for download on all major podcasting platforms.

In your own words, what exactly is "community pharmacy" as a niche profession?

I believe community pharmacy has a lot of untapped opportunities to make its transition into a tech-savvy world. Amazon and Alexa are spaces for pharmacy to enter into tele-health. There are changes going on in the community, such as Medication Therapy Management (MTM), that are allowing pharmacists to take on a more clinical role. Also, gaining provider status will allow pharmacists to practice at top of their setting. There is a large volume of patients for us to access and impact.

What was your role as a community pharmacist?

I started off floating as a community pharmacist. Four months later, I was promoted to the position of pharmacy manager. I started performing MTM at my store and showed the benefits of the program and that it was possible to incorporate into the community workflow. The district manager then sent a pharmacist to cover my shift once a week so I could work on MTM for different stores in my district. I would interact with patients on the phone and in person. Both the volume of patients and quality of work made me stand out. I went on to become a CDE (certified diabetes educator). Having a CDE is not necessary in community setting, but it opened up doors. I kept up with literature and was comfortable with reaching out to patients and doctors. I knew MTM would eventually lead to practicing in a clinical setting. In school, I knew I wanted as many doors open as possible, but I was unsure of exactly what I wanted to do at graduation.

Why do you enjoy contributing to the profession through this specialty? Tell us what gets you excited about your work!

I am a very competitive person and I am always wanting the next mountain to climb up. Medicine and healthcare are always changing, and I enjoy working and always learning.

What are the current requirements/certifications to practice in the community niche as a pharmacist?

Currently, the requirements to work in a community pharmacy are to have a PharmD, and many older pharmacists have a RPh. To get stuck in community pharmacy would be to not go after additional knowledge or courses to keep up on medicine. In order to make appropriate recommendations to patients, you need to be up to date on the medication evidence and guidelines.

If you could go back to your first day of pharmacy school, and knew that you would end up in community pharmacy, what steps would you take to build your professional résumé to best align you for success?

I did not always enjoy school, and I was not involved in extracurricular activities, because I worked a lot. I want to say I would be more involved, and one barrier I had in school was not wanting to do things the cookie-cutter way that things were taught. I was told I was different in my way of thinking. This led me to become more involved as a pharmacist. My recommendations to pharmacy students in order to stand out is to have a good work ethic, find out what you want out of your rotations, and have a desire to learn in a way that is impactful for future patient care.

What organizations, publications, or establishments would you recommend to follow to build a strong repertoire and/or better familiarize yourself with being an effective pharmacist in the community niche?

National Community Pharmacists Association (NCPA) is a good organization for those interested in community pharmacy. I recommend keeping up to date on literature by automating the process and signing up for free applications such as Medscape or Evidence Alerts. Also, getting email alerts from these resources will help to keep your continued learning time efficient.

Are there any suggestions you would make to a first-year pharmacy student to better prepare them or give them a good overview, or glimpse, if you will, into the "real world" of community pharmacy?

I recommend going through classes to make the most out of material and understand why all of your classes matter. Even classes many pharmacy students feel are unnecessary to their career goals, such as biochemistry and microbiology, are helpful with fully understanding pharmacology. You never know what you're going to be doing in the future and everything may be important. Opportunities open up with the people you might meet and it is important to reach out to people.

What have you found to be the best strategy for performing "deep work"—that is, focused time spent to efficiently produce quality results to advance your career?

I focus better at night when it's quiet and dark out, but this is different for everyone. I get coffee and caffeine, set time aside to get stuff done, and don't procrastinate. I finish projects as quick as I can so I can move onto my next project.

What overall suggestions would you make to become poised in the community niche of the profession of pharmacy throughout a student's time in pharmacy school?

To make yourself stand out as a student, you should ask for more responsibility and make yourself available to work on breaks. Learn from as many people as you can. Volunteer your time, shadow, and seek out good opportunities to learn and make a name for yourself. Be seriously passionate about wanting to be a great pharmacist.

Many thanks to Dr. Mike Corvino for his time in sharing his expertise on his roles, responsibilities, and best-practice tips in the specialty niche of pharmacy, and for student pharmacist Casey Butrus, who led this interview.

COMMUNITY PHARMACY II

Richard Waithe PharmD

President, VUCA Health; Founder of R_xRadio

Dr. Richard Waithe is passionate about helping people better manage their health and medications. While still in pharmacy school, Dr. Waithe played a key role on the content team as a junior editor in helping VUCA Health create the largest library of medication education videos. Fast forward to present day, as president, he is committed to continuing VUCA Health's mission of improving health literacy through increased access to reliable and understandable medication information.

With multiple leadership roles in community pharmacies that include Target, CVS, and Publix Pharmacy, and an innate ability to connect and engage with his patients, Richard has extensive experience in delivering quality medication therapy management services to help patients improve health outcomes. Dr. Waithe is also the Founder of R_xRadio, a digital media platform focused on engaging and inspiring pharmacists to better the profession of pharmacy. Through podcasting and producing media content for platforms like Facebook, Instagram, Alexa, LinkedIn, and Medium, R_xRadio quickly became an emerging leader in the digital media landscape of healthcare.

Richard received his Bachelor of Science in Chemistry from Florida International University and his Doctor of Pharmacy from the University of Florida.

In your own words, what exactly is "community pharmacy" as a niche profession?

Community pharmacy is going through an interesting period. I would call it a niche that has no barrier. Working in the community requires a special type of person to succeed. The day-to-day tasks are stressful and hard. Currently, the role of the pharmacist is largely dealing with inventory and dispensing. However, it is moving towards medication therapy management and focusing on clinical services due to recent improvements of technology and automation. Introducing automation into community pharmacy is expensive at the moment. However, when automation becomes more prevalent, it will open up more time for pharmacists to provide these clinical services to patients.

What was your role as a community pharmacist?

Working in community pharmacy as a pharmacist, my daily tasks included ensuring the patients were getting safe and effective medications. This included verifying prescriptions, checking for drug-drug interactions, taking action to call doctors, and working interprofessionally with other healthcare providers. A large part of the job is connecting with the patient and building a relationship. For patients who are not as receptive, it is the pharmacist's responsibility to make the patient aware of their health and the risks and benefits associated with their medication regimen. My job also included managing inventory and running a team. There is a large business aspect to community pharmacy. A community pharmacist is not expected to know everything. However, they do have a role in earning the trust of the patient as a credible healthcare professional and the pharmacist needs to know where and how to access the answer to medical questions quickly. A community pharmacist needs to be confident in their skills and knowledge.

Why do you enjoy contributing to the profession through this specialty? Tell us what gets you excited about your work!

Currently, I am the president of a company called VUCA Health. Our company focuses on creating healthcare content with videos, and there is account management with this business. We provide medication education videos to independent and chain pharmacies, hospitals, and health plans. We cover ninety percent of things commonly dispensed in the pharmacy. Although this differs from the traditional role of a community pharmacist, and is taking a step away from practicing with patients, there is still a large engagement with outreaching to patients on a population basis. I enjoy working for VUCA Health because I am reaching so many more patients now.

What are the current requirements/certifications to practice in the community niche as a pharmacist?

Currently, there is a low barrier to entry for pharmacy students. All that is required to work in most community settings is a PharmD. Residency is also an option but not necessary to work in the community. Some residencies may be beneficial for a student to consider depending on their career goals. A community pharmacist needs to have good leadership qualities and good soft skills of interacting and being personable with patients. For advancing in community pharmacy, it is not always about who you know, but how you can prove yourself as a leader.

If you could go back to your first day of pharmacy school, and knew that you would end up in community pharmacy, what steps would you take to build your professional résumé to best align you for success?

Going back, I would reach out to as many independent community pharmacies in the area where I want to live and begin helping them around the pharmacy and asking questions to improve their business model. For a pharmacy student, this builds a skill set and a good understanding of pharmacy as a business. Independent pharmacies are a great place to practice since there is more freedom for the pharmacy staff due to less bureaucracy.

What organizations, publications, or establishments would you recommend to follow to build a strong repertoire and/or better familiarize yourself with being an effective pharmacist in the community niche?

I recommend listening to my podcast $R_X Radio$. Other resources and organizations that are beneficial for prospective community pharmacists are Pharmacists Letter, APhA, and NASP. Pharmacists Letter provides good up-to-date information about what you need to know and changes that are occurring. NASP focuses on specialty pharmacy, which is a pivot from community pharmacy, but definitely a growing field of pharmacy.

Are there any suggestions you would make to a first-year pharmacy student to better prepare them or give them a good overview, or glimpse, if you will, into the "real world" of community pharmacy?

I would recommend getting first-hand experience working in a community pharmacy as early as possible. That is the only way to really experience what it is like to work in the real world of community pharmacy. Many things seen in the community pharmacy cannot be taught in school.

What have you found to be the best strategy for performing "deep work"—that is, focused time spent to efficiently produce quality results to advance your career?

I think this is more of a personal question to do what makes you happy and setting goals of what you want out of your career.

What overall suggestions would you make to become poised in the community niche of the profession of pharmacy throughout a student's time in pharmacy school?

Becoming self-aware of what you really want to do in pharmacy and actually doing that. The technology and roles of a pharmacist are developing in a way that it is possible to have a dream job. Students should always seek out new opportunities that they want for themselves. If that opportunity is not available, they should try to see if it would be possible to implement it themselves. It is not the end all to be all to complete a residency and there are still many opportunities for pharmacists who do not do a residency.

Any final thoughts?

For pharmacy students, I recommend also reading my book *First Time Pharmacist* to help prepare you for success. The future of pharmacy is leaning towards technology.

Amazon Alexa and voice applications and devices are going to be synonymous about how we use our phones right now. Using voice technology would be faster and more efficient for the patient to access information about their health. Pharmacists are already considered a trusted and accessible healthcare provider, and are already seeing roles in implementing voice technology to better patient care. We should use skill sets to work with technology. I don't see pharmacists being replaced by technology anytime in the near future. Google already exists and didn't replace pharmacists. The medical information is out there and patients have access to that at their fingertips. Although robots may take over the dispensing role of a technician, the cognitive abilities of a clinician that requires building emotional connection with patients is irreplaceable.

Many thanks to Dr. Richard Waithe for his time in sharing his expertise on his roles, responsibilities, and best-practice tips in the specialty niche of pharmacy, and for student pharmacist Casey Butrus, who led this interview.

RESIDENCY

Heather Johnson, PharmD, BCPS
Assistant Professor, Pharmacy and Therapeutics
University of Pittsburgh School of Pharmacy

Dr. Johnson is an Assistant Professor and Clinical Specialist in Transplantation at the University of Pittsburgh School of Pharmacy. She received her PharmD degree from the University of Minnesota College of Pharmacy in 1995, after which she completed a Clinical Fellowship in Renal Transplant Pharmacotherapy at Hennepin County Medical Center in Minneapolis, Minnesota. Dr. Johnson has been a member of the School of Pharmacy faculty since August 1997 and is a Board Certified Pharmacotherapy Specialist.

Dr. Johnson is a Clinical Specialist in the Transplant ICU at UPMC Presbyterian Shadyside where she works with members of transplant surgery and critical care medicine. Before joining the ICU, Dr. Johnson developed practices in ambulatory kidney transplant and viral hepatitis, and designed and implemented a pharmacy service in Palermo, Italy. Currently, her primary teaching focus is in liver disease and nutrition, but she also participates in the immunology course. Dr. Johnson's research interests are in the area of transplantation and pharmacokinetics in transplantation and liver disease.

Specific to this chapter on pursuing the residency track following pharmacy school, Dr. Johnson precepts both University of Pittsburgh Pharmacy students and pharmacy residents on clinical rotations in the Transplant ICU and is Director of the Transplant Pharmacy Residency (PGY2). In addition, Dr. Johnson coordinates a rotation for pharmacy students at ISMETT (the Mediterranean Institute for Specialized Therapy and Transplantation) in Palermo, Italy.

In your own words, what is the difference between the PharmD degree and pursuing a residency afterward? What values and benefits can a residency provide?

Residency gives you more opportunity to actually interact with other providers. This is not able to be simulated well enough just in pharmacy school. Residents get the opportunity to work with a variety of other healthcare professionals.

In school, there are a limited number of patient experiences with the primary goal being learning. Residency is vice versa in that patient care is the primary goal while you learn along the way. Residency is not as much of a simulation.

What is your role in assisting pharmacists and students in choosing a residency? What does that process look like?

My first objective is to understand what a student's goals are after residency and then help them choose based upon this. I help students to understand what kind of medical center or community pharmacy would be best to meet their career goals. For example, for those who want to specialize (PGY2), the academic medical center is typically the best area to go. The patient population within the center is also important.

Similar experiences are to be had at academic hospitals versus community hospitals, but there are differences. Oftentimes, those in community hospitals have more autonomy than those in academic centers.

What would you suggest for someone who is looking to choose a residency? What best constitutes a successful process?

Differentiate yourself by becoming active in organizations in pharmacy school early on, take on projects, demonstrate that you are a leader, and demonstrate that you are willing to teach and engage the next generation. Engage not only within curricular activities but also volunteerism and professional advocacy are important. Special projects, such as research, show that a student is willing to go above and beyond and is willing to take responsibility to be independent and develop a project that isn't necessarily well-defined in the beginning. Grades are good, but a 4.0 in the absence of any other engagement is not good because you do not know anything more about the applicant other than they studied a lot.

The interview: are there any "do's" and "don'ts" that applicants should be aware of?

You need to be able to answer the questions you are asked, to tell your story, and to tell why you want to be the pharmacist you want to be. Use examples that showcase the qualities that you think a resident should have, such as hard-working, kind, and good clinical judgement. Different programs are looking for different attributes. Most programs look for good time management skills.

Do not be negative about anything that you have done, including classes or others with whom you have worked. You want to be memorable but not in a bad way. Do not swear.

Why do you enjoy contributing to the profession through this specialty? Tell us what gets you excited about your work!

When I can add something that only the pharmacist could contribute and use my knowledge base to help a patient or provider. I enjoy being able to use my pharmacist-specific knowledge to aid the team such that patient care is improved. I appreciate feedback from patients, students, and professionals alike.

With residency, the fun part is how much the residents develop over the whole year. They have learned how to solve problems, handle a variety of patients, and think differently in general. In the beginning of residency, they go looking for an answer, much like they are still a student, but in the end, they learn that they have to come up with a response, which is different than an answer. Responses include monitoring and side effects, for example.

What are the current requirements or certifications are needed to qualify for a residency after the PharmD program—what does it take?

For most residencies, you have to be graduating from an ACPE-accredited program and be eligible for licensure in the state that you are pursuing as a residency. You must be able to practice as a pharmacist. It is the standard for PGY1 that the incoming resident be licensed within ninety days. Not all programs require immunizing status, but some do—typically ambulatory care or community residencies.

If you were a student who knew you were going to pursue a residency, and could go back to your first day of pharmacy school, what steps would you take to build your professional résumé to best align you for success?

I would find organizations that have opportunities for professional development as well as community service. It would be optimal to take on leadership roles in the organizations and hope to become involved in state or national versions of those organizations. I would also seek to attend their conferences. I would recommend seeking out volunteer experiences that are communication- and people-related. It would we beneficial to pursue a special topic as early as possible and do your best to make it longitudinal. I encourage getting a job, especially in a setting that you eventually might like to work. You will want to be thoughtful about the classes you take, but take as many that you can to diversify. I would also encourage you to engage with people who are not in your own class, especially upperclassmen so you can learn what steps are ahead of you so you can work ahead. You also have the opportunity to develop relationships with current residents and current pharmacists, who are a great source of knowledge.

What organizations, publications, or establishments would you recommend to follow to build a strong repertoire and better familiarize yourself with to successfully match a top choice in a pharmacy residency?

It depends on what you want to do. If you want to go after a community-based residency, APhA and PPA in Pennsylvania would be best. AMCP is best for managed care. If you are leaning toward a hospital-based practice, SCCP and SSHP are best. In Pennsylvania, there has been a stronger presence of SSHP versus SCCP, but other states are the opposite. Both of these have opportunities for students to be leaders on a national level, which is a great experience. Do not be afraid to reach for things like this! In general, the organizations have great resources that are good for residency preparation. Doing things like a patient counseling competition and clinical skills competition are very valuable for preparing for the field. Put all relevant experiences on your CV, including competitions, even if you did not win.

Are there any suggestions you would make to a first-year pharmacy student to better prepare them with a good overview, or glimpse, if you will, into the "real world" of the residency track? What would you say are some truths or expectations that may take some students by surprise that they might not expect as a resident that would help them feel more prepared had they known what to expect ahead of time?

Asking questions is extremely important, even for current students or residents. You need to make sure to take every opportunity to learn about all the options out there before it is too late. Expect the best and prepare for the worst. Don't limit your choices by having limited your preparation.

As far as surprises, people are often surprised by how much patient care is involved. It is a practice experience versus a learning experience. There is no watching involved, it is all doing.

What have you found to be the best strategy for performing "deep work"—that is, focused time spent to efficiently produce quality results to advance your career?

Structuring blocks of time and just dedicating it to one specific task is an effective strategy. Make sure that there are no other things during this time that could get in the way. It can be a short period of time and still be efficient.

What overall suggestions would you make to become poised in the profession of pharmacy as a residency candidate throughout pharmacy school?

Do as many things as you can do well such that you do not sacrifice grades for involvement, but the same goes for the other way around. When you get involved in a professional organization, you develop a lot of skills that are useful, like public speaking, communication, and patient care.

Any final thoughts?

What you think you are going to do when you finish your education and training is not usually what you will end up doing down the line. You need to be open to the idea of new things because you grow that way and the field of pharmacy is changing very quickly.

How did you end up at The University of Pittsburgh School of Pharmacy?

I ended up at Pitt because transplant was what I liked, but I actually discovered it by accident. The kidney is an important organ, and my program offered some nephrology rotations, but I did not resonate with the instructor who precepted those rotations. I chose transplant instead within the nephrology division such that I could get exposure to kidneys without doing the rotation with this instructor.

In the transplant rotation, I got the opportunity to work on the inpatient side within the clinic and on the ambulatory side and loved that I was able to be a part of my patients' care every step of the way. I applied to the residency position that was in the same unit as my rotation. After being accepted, I cancelled my other residency interviews and said I wanted to stay.

At the time I finished my residency, there were not many job opportunities available in transplant pharmacy. There were options in New Orleans, Madison, Wisconsin, and Pitt. I liked Pittsburgh the most and came here when I was given the job offer. I came here to do ambulatory kidney transplant both on inpatient and outpatient side.

On the inpatient side, I was noticing dosage problems with a lot of the patients' medications, so I asked if I could start rounding with the inpatient kidney service. From this, I was able to develop a program of rounding with physicians in transplant at the University of Pittsburgh Medical Center (UPMC). UPMC then developed a program in Italy, and I volunteered and made my case to go based on my creation of the rounding program at UPMC Presbyterian. I was approved to go and developed the pharmacy program in Palermo, Italy, and lived there for six years. I then came back to Pittsburgh to be a liver transplant ICU pharmacist at UPMC Presbyterian. I did not end up at all where I thought I would. All along the way, I was always involved in developing something new. Always be open to new opportunities.

Many thanks to Dr. Heather Johnson for her time in sharing her expertise on his roles, responsibilities, and best-practice tips in the specialty niche of pharmacy, and for student pharmacist Dan Schrum, who led this interview.

BUSINESS IN PHARMACY

Gordon J. Vanscoy, PharmD, CACP, MBA

Associate Dean for Business Innovation, Associate Professor, Pharmacy and Therapeutics, University of Pittsburgh School of Pharmacy

Dr. Gordon J. Vanscoy possesses over two and a half decades of executive experience in the healthcare industry, creating and leading successful medical/pharmaceutical service business ventures. He is the managing partner of Relentless Capital, a health technology angel investment firm; he is chairman & CEO of PANTHER$_x$ Specialty Pharmacy; and chairman of OTCme and GreenCAR$_x$E. Dr. Vanscoy also is the Associate Dean for Business Innovation and Associate Professor of Pharmacy and Therapeutics at the University of Pittsburgh.

While Dr. Vanscoy was Pitt's former Assistant Dean for Managed Care, he rose in the private sector to Executive Vice President and Chief Operating Officer of the nation's first specialty pharmacy—Stadtlander Operating Company—which was sold to Counsel Corporation. He then moved to AmeriSource Bergen Specialty Group and ultimately CVS ProCare. As Vice-Chair of the Department of Pharmacy and Therapeutics, he was the founding director of the University of Pittsburgh Medical Center's Drug Information and Pharmacoepidemiology Center. He was also an active member of the University Biomedical Institutional Review Board, serving as vice chairman for a period of time. Prior to that, and as founding director, Dr. Vanscoy developed the country's first Anticoagulation Clinic Service and obtained prescribing privileges at the Pittsburgh Veterans Affairs Health System.

Dr. Vanscoy received his Bachelor of Science in Pharmacy and Masters of Business Administration degrees from the University of Pittsburgh and his Doctor of Pharmacy degree from Duquesne University. He has completed an ASHP-accredited clinical residency and a fellowship in geriatrics. Dr. Vanscoy is a Certified Anticoagulation Care Provider.

His primary research interests include economic modeling of high-risk, high-cost disease states related to oncology, cardiology, critical care, and anticoagulation. His scholarly focus is on advancing education in entrepreneurship and the business of medicines to create future leaders.

Dr. Vanscoy has published a number of textbook chapters, more than two hundred scientific papers, and has received dozens of research grants and awards. In 2002, Dr. Vanscoy received the National Leadership Award from the Republican Congressional Committee Business Advisory Council. He was a finalist for the Ernst & Young Entrepreneur of the Year Award Western Pennsylvania Region in 2004. Gordon was recognized as Alumnus of the Year in 2008 by the University of Pittsburgh School of Pharmacy. He has provided more than seven hundred invited lectures and has served on many national and international committees. He is a past member of the International Society of Pharmaceutical Outcomes (ISPOR) Board of Directors, and the United States Pharmacopoeia's (USP) Therapeutic Information Management Advisory Panel. Gordon founded the credentialing body titled the National Certified Anticoagulation Care Providers, where he remains on the Board of Directors. In 2010, Dr. Vanscoy completed his term second term as Chairman of the Board of Directors of the American Red Cross Westmoreland County Chestnut Ridge Chapter.

In your own words, what exactly is pharmacy business as a niche profession?

Every aspect of pharmacy has a component of business; it is not a true specialty. So many aspects where we look at providing a service or product require business fundamentally because we need to be payed or reimbursed. We use the language of clinical pharmacy to move away from business, but it made us lose sight and not get paid or have our value recognized by society. Recently, they have started embracing business and getting paid for the value added. It is important to see business in every aspect of pharmacy.

What is your role as a pharmacist in business?

At this point, I am a leader and mentor. I train teams and am able to survey and identify opportunities. I lead people and organizations to find success. My work as a mentor is most enjoyable, the caffeine in my day. I give young people insight, catalyzing their career and helping them succeed at a faster rate.

Why do you enjoy contributing to the profession through this specialty? Tell us what gets you excited about your work!

As a leader, I enjoy creating new services, businesses, and approaches to solving problems. I get bored easily and have needed to transition into a new role every five years. I like to not follow the pack, but explore new, unique ways of doing things. I also am excited about giving back by mentoring people and institutions that have helped me along my own journey. I like to see others benefit from my experiences.

What are the current requirements or certifications to practice in a business setting of pharmacy?

For individuals, there are none that are necessary, but organizations need accreditations to get payers. If a student wants to have a way to differentiate him or herself, they can purse classes in accounting or law. They are trying to make new ways to accelerate the learning such as MBA programs, residencies, and the new Master of Science in Pharmacy Business Administration (MSPBA), a collaborative program at the University of Pittsburgh between the School of Pharmacy and the Joseph M. Katz Graduate School of Business. These may all help, but experience is most important.

If you could go back to your first day of pharmacy school, and knew that you would end up in business, what steps would you take to build your professional résumé to best align you for success?

I would take the executive lecture series course that Pitt offers to its students. However, not a single person knows exactly what they will do, so many CEOs simply find multiple opportunities. If one path does not work, you need to branch off, but everything you do contributes to your experience—no time is lost or wasted. So, work hard at whatever you are doing. The key is to be relentless. Some people have extreme talent and intelligence, but they also need ambition and relentlessness. It is also important to have great interpersonal skills. Never have one strategy or path—always look at other opportunities. Plans are good because they make you think and focus, but sticking to them can stifle your career.

What organizations, publications, or establishments would you recommend to follow to build a strong repertoire and better familiarize yourself with the field of business?

There is nothing unique about the pharmacy business, so become familiar with industry and business in general. Most prominent C-seat pharmacy business positions are filled by people outside of pharmacy. You need them to recognize you as a business person and not a skilled technician like many business people look at pharmacists. Some ways to familiarize yourself with business are using Twitter and following the *Wall Street Journal*, *New York Times*, and local news. Social media has made it much more efficient to stay informed. I recommend some books also. *Becoming Your Best* by Steven Shallenberger, *How to be a Positive Leader* by Jane Dutton and Gretchen Spreitzer, and *You Win in the Locker Room First* by John Gordon and Mike Smith.

Are there any suggestions you would make to a first-year pharmacy student to better prepare them or give them a good overview, or glimpse, if you will, into the "real world" of the business side of pharmacy?

Find a mentor you respect in a position you like, a position of authority. One of mine was my father and I had two others during my career. You can develop a relationship with a mentor, build trust, receive advice, and it helps you more than you know. You start to recognize attributes that you want to emulate.

What overall suggestions would you make to become poised in the profession of pharmacy throughout pharmacy school?

Don't be afraid to fail, as not all businesses succeed. It is a bitter pill to swallow, but you learn more from failure. When you graduate, everyone looks like you so, make sure you differentiate yourself. Constantly update your CV. Make sure that people have a good perception of you because opportunities are presented to you because of who or what you are. Be relentless, now is the time to put in the extra effort.

What are the biggest hurdles to expect when you start out as an entrepreneur, and what suggestions would you give when they are encountered to overcome them? Any final thoughts?

Getting over fear of risk. There is always risk, whether it is financial or a failure, that may impact your reputation. And, you just have to accept the risk. Also, do not be shy about promoting yourself and your business. Be a salesman. Realize that no one has the entire skill set to be successful—you have to do introspection and see your weaknesses. Then, surround yourself with those who can complement your deficiencies. You need an entire team.

If it was easy, everyone would do it.

Many thanks to Dr. Gordon J. Vancscoy for his time in sharing his expertise on his roles, responsibilities, and best-practice tips in the specialty niche of pharmacy, and for student pharmacist Heather Johnson, who led this interview.

DIABETES CARE/CERTIFIED DIABETES EDUCATOR (CDE)

Scott R. Drab, PharmD, CDE, BC-ADM
Associate Professor, Pharmacy and Therapeutics,
University of Pittsburgh School of Pharmacy

Dr. Scott Drab is an Associate Professor of Pharmacy & Therapeutics and Director of University Diabetes Care Associates. He received his Bachelor of Science degree in Pharmacy from the University of Pittsburgh and his Doctor of Pharmacy degree from Duquesne University.

Dr. Drab's efforts contributing to pharmaceutical care led to the creation of one of the first pharmacist-run diabetes care centers located in a community independent pharmacy. As a Certified Diabetes Educator and director of the clinic, he is responsible for care plan development, education, and patient follow-up. He has managed the care of hundreds of diabetic patients over the years, improving clinical health outcomes. In addition to direct patient care responsibilities, Dr. Drab is responsible for providing drug information to the surrounding medical community and provides outreach education to benefit the greater good of the community. Today, University Diabetes Care Associates serves as a model and prototype for future care centers.

Dr. Drab's teaching responsibilities at the school of pharmacy involve clinical instruction as well as classroom teaching. His classes are centered on collaborative and inquiry-based learning while he strives to provide a classroom environment that simulates the practice environment.

Dr. Drab currently serves on several school and university committees, including the Experiential Learning Committee, Academic Performance Committee, Pharm D Council, University Senate Community Relations Committee, and the Pitt Pathway Committee. He also serves as faculty advisor and liaison between students and the

National Community Pharmacists Association.

He has received the Roche Preceptor of the Year Award in 2003 and 2008 and was selected as the 2007 Recipient of the Pennsylvania Society of Health System Pharmacist's Joe E. Smith Award. The Joe E. Smith award is awarded to a member of PSHP, who demonstrates excellence in practice, and is deserving of recognition for service to his institution, community, and the profession.

In your own words, what exactly is diabetes care as a niche profession?

Training, education, and helping patients to achieve their desired outcomes would be the simplest way to define diabetes care—it's all about the patient.

What is your role as a pharmacist in diabetes management?

As the owner of the University Diabetes Care Associates Clinic, I serve as the diabetes educator and director of the clinic. We serve to treat and see patients to really help them understand diabetes, and to optimize their outcomes in working with them as an advocate for their best health.

The clinic itself is a clinical teaching facility for both students on rotation and residents to grow their skills in diabetes-centered care for patients.

Why do you enjoy contributing to the profession through this specialty? Tell us what gets you excited about your work!

From a patient care perspective, when patients come in and they are unfamiliar, or do not have the knowledge surrounding diabetes or diabetes care, it is rewarding seeing that when they leave they have the knowledge to better take care of themselves.

From a pharmacy student perspective, training students who don't have a great understanding of diabetes and helping them through that so that when they finally learn and understand the disease, they can then help and teach patients and other students with the experience they gained from this site.

For me, the teaching of students is the biggest contribution to the field of pharmacy. I enjoy mentoring both groups of students and one-on-one to really go in-depth to explore and develop the skills they have so that they can then give that back to their patients.

What are the current requirements or certifications to practice in a diabetes education setting?

In Pennsylvania, there are none specifically as of now, however, the state is thinking about licensing diabetes educators. I highly recommend becoming a certified diabetes educator (CDE) or board certified in advanced diabetes management (BCADM). Please note that other states do have licensing requirements based on where you practice.

If you could go back to your first day of pharmacy school, and knew that you would end up in diabetes care, what steps would you take to build your professional résumé to best align you for success?

I would have sought out more shadowing and volunteer experiences. I would have also become more involved in the American Diabetes Association (ADA). Earlier engagement in diabetes, such as courses or electives offered, would have really benefited me earlier in my career path. When I was in pharmacy school, there was only one elective offered and it was in pharmacokinetics.

What organizations, publications, or establishments would you recommend to follow to build a strong repertoire and better familiarize yourself with the field of diabetes care?

The American Diabetes Association and its publication *Diabetes Care*. They also publish *Diabetes*, which is another good resource.

There is also American Association of Diabetes Educators (AADE).

Worth noting is an exceptional resource for pharmacy students who would highly benefit from if they are looking to really develop their skills in diabetes. If I was a student looking to learn more about diabetes, and how to provide optimal care for patients, DM Educate is the elective course offered at the School of Pharmacy. The great thing about this course is that it can be taken online, and is a good way to get involved in diabetes education, as any pharmacy student can take it.

[Editor's Note: I (Adam) have taken and helped to develop this course. It is without a doubt the simplest and most effective learning resource available to build a strong foundation and advance your skills in diabetes care. Highly recommended—see the Resources section at the end of this book for more information on this free course!]

Are there any suggestions you would make to a first-year pharmacy student to better prepare them or give them a good overview, or glimpse, if you will, into the "real world" of diabetes care?

I recommend that you interact with patients at their pharmacy who have diabetes, and learn as much as you can about diabetes. Make sure you understand the basic anatomy/physiology related to diabetes, as most of what diabetes is revolves around what was learned in the P1 year of pharmacy school.

What overall suggestions would you make to become poised in the profession of pharmacy focusing on diabetes care throughout pharmacy school?

Start with any educational opportunities that exist related to diabetes: continuing education lectures, organizational meetings, whatever it is, take advantage of the learning! You don't necessarily need to take elaborate courses, but start off taking small continuing education courses on diabetes medications, then slowly progress to medical continuing education.

What have you found to be the best strategy for performing "deep work"—that is, focused time spent to efficiently produce quality results to advance your career?

You need to find time—not in the clinic, not with patients, not being sought after by student or physicians—but time to yourself. Make this a priority to find as much time to yourself as you possibly can.

Any final thoughts?

I recommend that you start with basic diabetes education and continuing education courses, then build up the number of courses that you take. Overall, try to take every diabetes learning opportunity that exists, no matter how small. The most impactful opportunity you can create is to shadow a professional. If you get involved in working with someone in the diabetes field, this will really help you a lot.

Many thanks to Dr. Scott Drab for his time in sharing his expertise on his roles, responsibilities, and best-practice tips in the specialty niche of pharmacy, and for student pharmacist Maria Langas, who led this interview.

RESEARCH I

Pamela L. Smithburger, PharmD, MS, BCPS, BCCCP, FCCP

Associate Professor, Pharmacy and Therapeutics,
University of Pittsburgh School of Pharmacy

Dr. Pamela L. Smithburger earned her PharmD from the University of Pittsburgh School of Pharmacy. Upon graduation, she completed an ASHP-accredited Pharmacy Practice Residency and an ASHP-accredited Critical Care Specialty Residency at the University of Pittsburgh Medical Center. Dr. Smithburger has also completed the Master of Science Program in Clinical Research from the University of Pittsburgh School of Medicine.

Dr. Smithburger's clinical practice site is the Medical Intensive Care Unit at the University of Pittsburgh Medical Center, Presbyterian Hospital. She works closely with the physicians in the Pulmonology/Critical Care unit, and with nurses and other healthcare professionals to optimize medication therapies for patients requiring specialized care. Dr. Smithburger precepts pharmacy students during their experiential learning component of the Doctor of Pharmacy Program, as well as Pharmacy Practice and Critical Care Specialty residents in the UPMC residency program.

She is the program director for the Critical Care Residency and teaches in various courses throughout the PharmD curriculum, primarily focusing on disease states and drug therapy for the critically ill patient population. Dr. Smithburger's research focus is patient safety in the ICU as well as sedation and delirium management.

In your own words, what exactly is pharmacy research as a niche profession?

Research based in clinical practice is a way to help answer questions that you see clinically with patients for whom you feel having solutions can improve care, safety, or both. My research breaks off from these questions and unanswered topics in the clinical setting.

What is your role as a pharmacist in research?

My role is to help drive best practices with optimizing therapy to improve patient outcomes and safety. I do this through identifying the need for practice and designing an investigation to best answer or provide additional evidence for a specific way to practice and/or use medications.

Why do you enjoy contributing to the profession through this specialty? Tell us what gets you excited about your work!

Watching the research or investigations I have conducted directly impact patients who I am caring for on a daily basis, as well as impacting patients on a larger scale, is what drives me. For example, the work I have done concerning delirium has been implemented across UPMC as a standard of care. I find it rewarding not just locally from improved care to my patients through the service I deliver, but also impacting patients on a more global scale (i.e., throughout all of the UPMC healthcare system). Helping other clinicians and other institutions incorporate best practices and give evidence and ideas of how to handle difficult situations is something I truly enjoy in my practice.

What are the current requirements or certifications to practice in a research setting?

To best practice in the research setting, it's best to have some formalized training, meaning at minimum completing a residency or fellowship training. A residency training sets the stage to conduct clinical research, but additional training helps to further specify and analyze research. In my own career path, I sought a master's degree in clinical research; this greatly helped me to conduct research as well as lead projects and do analysis associated with research projects. It also provided additional foundations to lead projects on a larger scale and to incorporate more complex methods and analyses.

What is your proudest work?

The development and implementation of a non-pharmacologic delirium protocol, and setting the ground work for a family-based delirium prevention protocol.

If you could go back to your first day of pharmacy school, and knew that you would end up in research, what steps would you take to build your professional résumé to best align you for success?

While I was in pharmacy school, there were not as many opportunities to personalize education. However, if I was starting as a pharmacy student now, I would get involved in Research ARCO and Pharmacotherapy Scholars. Experience is invaluable, so I would actively seek out research opportunities early in pharmacy school. Building connections would be a big priority, so I would email faculty and ask to set up a short meeting to talk with them and find out what their research interest is as well as what their program is like. A lot of students don't do this because they don't want to bother faculty, but we are excited about what we are doing, and we want to provide the experience for the students as much as possible! I highly recommend that you engage and talk with different faculty members about their research—specifically where they are currently, how they got there, and what their career path looked like.

What organizations, publications, or establishments would you recommend to follow to build a strong repertoire and better familiarize yourself with the field of research?

In pharmacy, the American College of Clinical Pharmacists (ACCP) has a strong research network. Within ACCP, the Pharmacy Based Research Network (PBRN) provides training and other information for research and is a strong clinical/research-based organization. Pharmacy students have access to PBRN as long as you are a member of ACCP.

Overall, the Practice Research Networks (PRNs) are specialties that offer abstract and travel awards for students to help travel to meetings, which can help offset potential financial barriers to networking and gaining more experience with research. I highly recommend this as it is a good avenue for pharmacy students to get involved in research and network! If you have a more specialized area of interest, look specifically for organizations in your interest area. For example, if you are looking into critical care, check out the Society of Critical Care Medicine.

Are there any suggestions you would make to a first-year pharmacy student to better prepare them or give them a good overview, or glimpse, if you will, into the "real world" of pharmacy research?

My best advice is to reach out to faculty to learn about projects and just get your feet wet! This can start small, through helping with a small piece of a project or shadowing a faculty member to see their clinical practice and how it fits into the overall practice and specialty of focus. You can start very early on in you pharmacy career, seeking opportunities to go on clinical rounds and do research as a P1, and then continue on to do a special topics elective later on in the curriculum.

What have you found to be the best strategy for performing "deep work"—that is, focused time spent to efficiently produce quality results to advance your career?

This is a difficult task because the position has so many responsibilities, but I am able to accomplish this by carving out time in my schedule and blocking off two to three hours in advance so time does not get scheduled over. As a student, it can be very difficult to balance everything at first, but my best advice would be for you to plan ahead of time and dedicate specific time to different priorities. My number one tip when it comes to time management is this: *do not over schedule!* Find balance to enjoy what you're doing, as you do not want it to become a chore and get a negative impression of research. Make sure you have the time to dedicate.

What overall suggestions would you make to become poised in the profession of pharmacy research throughout pharmacy school?

In school, identify your passion for research and develop basic skills. You will probably not become an expert during pharmacy school, but you can most certainly strengthen your foundation to excel as your career progresses. Effective ways to do this would be for you to get involved in projects and gain a wide range of experiences with research, e.g., pro- and retrospective, Investigational Review Board (IRB), data collection, and analysis, as this will equip you to see all phases of research! At Pitt Pharmacy, we have the option for you to pursue Special Topics and Research ARCO.

After you graduate pharmacy school, ensure the residency you match with has a strong track record of publishing scholarly research projects or a research series to give you foundation for research. You can also seek fellowship or another advanced degree in research, such as studying for a master's in clinical research.

Many thanks to Dr. Pamela Smithburger for her time in sharing his expertise on her roles, responsibilities, and best-practice tips in the specialty niche of pharmacy, and for student pharmacist Rebecca Wytiaz, who led this interview.

RESEARCH II

Olufunmilola Abraham, BPharm, PhD
Assistant Professor, Pharmacy and Therapeutics,
University of Pittsburgh School of Pharmacy

Dr. Olufunmilola Abraham is an Assistant Professor in the Department of Pharmacy and Therapeutics School of Pharmacy and the Clinical & Translational Science Institute (CTSI), University of Pittsburgh. She received her Bachelor of Pharmacy (BPharm) degree from University of Lagos, Nigeria. Dr. Abraham received her Master's of Science and Doctor of Philosophy in Social and Administrative Sciences in Pharmacy from the University of Wisconsin-Madison School of Pharmacy and a Doctor of Philosophy minor in the Department of Industrial and Systems Engineering, focused on Human Factors Engineering and Patient Safety.

Dr. Abraham is a health services researcher, whose program of research aims to enhance medication adherence, patient safety, and quality of care for vulnerable populations in the community. Her research centers on utilizing human factors and systems engineering approaches to design interventions that improve patient care in a variety of community settings, such as pharmacies, primary care clinics, faith-based organizations, and community centers. She partners with healthcare professionals in these settings to understand processes and technologies that impact medication safety, quality of care, and adherence to medications. She has been the principal investigator on several projects funded by the Community Pharmacy Foundation, the University of Pittsburgh CTSI, the Pennsylvania Pharmacists Association, and AcademyHealth.

Dr. Abraham's teaching and research interests revolve around three main areas: 1. enhancing pharmacists' understanding of the impact of health information technology on patient care, adherence, and medication safety; 2. equipping students with the skills to apply human factors and systems engineering concepts and techniques in health services research; and 3. providing pharmacists and students with tools and skills needed to care for vulnerable patient populations in the community, such as children, adolescents, and older adults.

In your own words, what exactly is pharmacy research as a niche profession?

Pharmacy research is looking at how medication use impacts people's lives and how pharmacists can participate in appropriate medication use. This kind of research shows how, as pharmacists, we are responsible for assisting patients with appropriate medication use.

What is your role as a pharmacist in research?

As a faculty member, I identify current and important research topics by initiating projects based off of the gaps in patient care. As a pharmacist in research, I am able to understand and work to improve the pharmacy profession, pharmacy practice, and the overall health of people.

Why do you enjoy contributing to the profession through this specialty? Tell us what gets you excited about your work!

I'm given the opportunity to innovate and think outside the box of where this profession can go. I have the liberty to think of what is missing, which gives me flexibility in the topics with which I work. I work with other faculty who are just as excited about what we are doing. Working with students who are intimidated by research and showing them the value of people-centered research excites me the most.

What are the current requirements or certifications to practice in a research setting?

There are not many specific requirements, but there are many opportunities to be involved as a student. Many of these opportunities are woven into the curriculum. When a student identifies where their passion meets their drive, that is when they will thrive. This will motivates them to do outside work and take extra steps to volunteer with faculty. This can prepare them for post-graduate residencies and fellowships that would qualify them to practice in a research setting.

If you could go back to your first day of pharmacy school, and knew that you would end up in research, what steps would you take to build your professional résumé to best align you for success?

I would work to find my passion early on in my training. I would then have identified a faculty mentor with whom my interests aligned, and shadowed their expertise. Residents who struggle with research may have missed out on the mentored research experience during school, so by doing this early on, it will set you far ahead in your field. I would make sure to gain writing and presenting research experience in a professional setting, such as a conference.

What organizations, publications, or establishments would you recommend to follow to build a strong repertoire and better familiarize yourself with the field of research?

American Pharmacist Association (APhA) and the *Journal of American Pharmacist Association* (JAPA) are great resources. The journal's audience is both researchers and practitioners. State organizations of pharmacy and non-pharmacy journals, such as physician and informatics-based journals, are another great option, as interprofessional work can improve medication safety and pharmacy practice.

Are there any suggestions you would make to a first-year pharmacy student to better prepare or give them a good overview, or glimpse, if you will, into the "real world" of pharmacy research?

In your first year of pharmacy school, identify a faculty member who you could learn from and work with them. When looking for a faculty member who you can learn from, do not be afraid to fail or to volunteer with someone.

What have you found to be the best strategy for performing "deep work"—that is, focused time spent to efficiently produce quality results to advance your career?

What has helped me the most is figuring out what I'm passionate about. Knowing what I'm passionate about gives me the internal drive necessary to complete a project. Finding the marriage between my passions and a need that people have has been the key. Personally, some of those "marriages" have included the opioid epidemic and medication safety and use in children.

What overall suggestions would you make to become poised in the profession of pharmacy research throughout pharmacy school?

Find mentors who are in tune with your needs, overlap in your research passion and interests, and who are invested in your career development.

Any final thoughts?

This is a really important book and I would like to be a co-author on it to share my experiences working with students over the past four years. I would like to show what works and what doesn't to help students thrive through the research process. Faculty should be able to put that first in any mentorship.

Many thanks to Dr. Olufunmilola Abraham for her time in sharing her expertise on her roles, responsibilities, and best-practice tips in the specialty niche of pharmacy, and for student pharmacist Kathy Monangai, who led this interview.

PHARMD TO PHD TRACK

Philip E. Empey, PharmD, PhD

Assistant Professor, Pharmacy and Therapeutics,
University of Pittsburgh School of Pharmacy

Dr. Philip Empey is the Associate Director for Pharmacogenomics of the Pitt/UPMC Institute of Precision Medicine and leads the PreCISE-R$_x$ and Test2Learn teams to implement pharmacogenomics clinical, research, and educational initiatives. As a clinician-scientist in the Department of Pharmacy and Therapeutics, Dr. Empey conducts NIH-funded clinical and translational research aimed at understanding the mechanisms of the variability in drug response to improve medication-related outcomes in critically ill patients.

Dr. Empey received his PharmD from the University of Rhode Island and completed PGY1 and PGY2 residencies in Pharmacy Practice and Critical Care at the University of Kentucky. He earned a Doctor of Philosophy in Clinical Pharmaceutical Sciences at the University of Kentucky before completing postdoctoral research training at the University of Pittsburgh.

Current research interests include understanding the role and impact of xenobiotic transporters following neurological injury, transporter pharmacogenomics, pharmacogenomics clinical implementation, collection of medication-related phenotype information, and genotype-phenotype discovery. Dr. Empey teaches at the graduate level in pharmacokinetics, pharmacogenomics, and drug transporters in the Schools of Pharmacy, Medicine, and Nursing at the University of Pittsburgh. He also has a research interest in innovative educational models to transform education.

In your own words, what is the difference between the PharmD degree and obtaining a PhD afterward? What are the values or benefits of a doctor of philosophy?

The PharmD degree is sort of the final preparatory degree to become a pharmacist. I think that going on to advanced research training is important if you want to be involved in completing research, lead research projects, if you want to contribute to the science of either drug use or drug utility, or any of those domains. Essentially, the PhD degree is a research-based degree. And it's a great additional training if you want to go into a specific field. With your pharmacist license, you need additional research-based training.

When it comes to the career path in earning a PhD after a PharmD, there are a couple different paths. If we have a lot of students who are interested in research, right in pharmacy school students can get involved in research by doing independent studies with faculty members. We have a program designed for this purpose called Special Topics right here at Pitt Pharmacy, but also you can go on to get areas of concentration in research. Some students go through special classes or do research projects with faculty members, and then students who want to go into more involved. Research experiences can occur either seeking a special research training during or after a PharmD degree. So it could be something like a research-based fellowship or a PhD. With that mention, fellowships have traditionally been a training path for folks who were interested in research. I would get a high level of clinical training and would want to learn a little bit of research on top of it. PhD degrees are the traditional degree of someone who wants to commit a significant amount of training to really make research the core of what they want to do in the future. So, if you look around the school, many of our faculty are trained through either path, but anyone who is really doing a significant part of their research in their future is beginning to become more rare than folks who wouldn't have some concentration in additional research training, as it's hard to run research groups and to conduct large clinical trial. That's a discipline, just like pharmacy training, that is somewhat special. This requires unique skills, a unique experience, and a PhD gives you the breadth and the depth of that training.

As far as the value or benefit that a PhD, in addition to a PharmD degree, it comes down to your focus and intent. For me, I'm a pharmacist in Pennsylvania, and I've gone through residency training, so I did that before I did a PhD track. But I knew very early on that I wanted to contribute to research and I wanted to be able to publish findings from trials from either clinical trials or preclinical trials that would advance the practice of pharmacy and medicine.

What is your role as a PhD in pharmacy?

Specifically, my main role in the pharmacy school was to always be in teaching and to lead a research team that conducts research to advance pharmacy and medicine, with my areas focusing in pharmacokinetics and pharmacogenomics. So, with the PhD training, I'm then also responsible for leading a group, writing grant proposals, designing research studies, and leading a team that's able to answer questions related to them. That means other students, pharmacists, researchers, technicians, data analysts, folks in medicine as well as in pharmacy, and even outside of any type of medical field, all coming together to answer these big research questions.

Why do you enjoy contributing to the profession through this specialty? Tell us what gets you excited about your work!

When I was a practicing pharmacist, I kept encountering questions to which I couldn't find answers. Why does this patient respond to this drug differently? We've prescribed this medication hundreds of times before, and this one had a side effect we didn't expect or this patient already has this other condition and we know it's going to interfere with the way the drug is cleared. How do we dose this patient? Some of those questions have answers by going to the package labeling or what we've learned in pharmacy school, but all too often I've found that the answers were not available. Then usually you go to the primary literature and read and try to find those studies, and sometimes you find a study that's close, but not quite done the right way to answer the question.

Scenarios like these can be really frustrating as a clinician, and I kept finding myself asking questions to which I couldn't find answers. Being in a position to try to ask, and actually try to solve those problems, is what really gets me excited. So, if someone asked me whether we should be conducting a pharmacogenomic testing in practice, we don't know what some of the outcomes may be or how easy it is to perform or whether it's even feasible in the health system. We're conducting that research to show that we can do it, that testing can be established, and what the impact on patient care is. We're actually able to drive changes in practice and we've already been able to see those changes. In this regard, we already have new practice models set up because we were able to show something in research. I think what's fun is that I can say something we've created in the lab, and researched and tested in the lab, has made its way to improve a patient's life.

What are the current requirements or certifications to obtain a PhD after the PharmD program—what does it take?

With the PhD program, there are incoming requirements. For our program here at Pitt Pharmacy, there actually aren't many incoming students who leave right after graduating with a PharmD from Pitt, or elsewhere, and come right into the PhD program. We actually had some students who don't even have a pharmacy degree, so what really makes for a good candidate to get PhD training is someone who's really passionate about research, wants to learn research techniques and be a leader in the field of research long term, and is really just committed to that—the research background and that future training. Now, obviously if someone has had the experience in research already, and really knows they want to work in a particular area with a particular person, it's helpful, but not all of our students know that coming into the program. I would say that those are the incoming requirements to be successful in the PhD program. We're looking for folks who just really have a passion to learn, who are independent thinkers, and like working in teams because research is a very collaborative thing. It actually is sometimes more collaborative than working in a pharmacy, as everyday we're working in large teams. Overall, if someone is passionate about advancing the field, those students can become successful and end up being the change agents for the future.

If you could go back to your first day of pharmacy school, and knew that you would end up pursuing a PhD in pharmacy, what steps would you take to build your professional résumé to best align you for success?

Looking back to my first day, I didn't know this was what I wanted to do, and, overall, most people don't know. That's the biggest thing—you learn through pharmacy school by getting a bunch of different experiences for what you like and don't like. This is a key concept that we tell students. You can personalize your education here at Pitt Pharmacy and many other pharmacy schools, but you absolutely should take advantage of the opportunities around you. I didn't realize that I liked research really until my third year of pharmacy school. I liked a faculty member who was teaching me pharmacokinetics in critical care, and I came up to him after he had made an announcement, "Anybody who wants to do research, come see me." I told him I think I might be interested. He welcomed me into the lab. At the end of that six weeks' time with him, I knew that I wanted that to be a part of my life sometime in the future, so from that point on, it was easier with that clarity for me to look for opportunities where I could learn more about research. So, the secret really is to explore your opportunities as much as possible. If you learn very quickly that you really hate something, like *I don't like research* or *I don't like working in a community setting,* or whatever, then it helps you narrow what you do like. It only gets harder as you go through pharmacy school. You can easily dabble when you are in pharmacy school, to do a research project for a semester, and then switch gears. But, if you already have a job and a family and a busy life after graduation, it becomes much harder to explore opportunities.

What organizations, publications, or establishments would you recommend to follow to build a strong repertoire and better familiarize yourself with earning a PhD in pharmacy?

My best advice is to learn about all the different programs and decide where to go. The University of Pittsburgh School of Pharmacy has a wonderful program that is very translational. It gets folks doing clinically-related projects that impact human health, but you really have to understand the landscape. Find your best fit so you end up at a program where you can get the experience you want from a training perspective, and you can work with folks who want you to learn the most. The biggest thing is to look around to get a sense of where the best fit for you might be. The other thing to do is to get as much experience as you can beforehand to help make that decision easier!

It's much harder to apply to places and to prepare for a PhD if you don't know what you want to do. We have had some students who come in and say, "I think I might like research." Well, you don't want to learn by applying to a PhD program. You're starting another full four- to five-year graduate degree and nobody wants anyone to make a bad decision. As soon as you gain an interest, get exposure, reach out to faculty members in the school, and start exploring—especially here at Pitt Pharmacy. Their doors are always open for you. You can get involved in different types of research, whether it's research in the clinical setting, using the electronic health record, the community setting, in the lab, or computer-based research. You can even work preclinically in the cell culture, in animals for example, or doing computation that will help the team to design drugs in the medical chemistry roles. They're all available, and faculty are doing those types of research every day.

My research was originally, and still is, focused on pharmacokinetics, and that is pretty broad. We basically determine how a drug moves throughout the body and anything that affects it. We may look at how clinical factors like critical care or an illness or a trauma affect how your drug is eliminated. Also, things like genetics, as genetic disposition may make you more or less responsive to a medication or more likely to have a side effect.

There is not one umbrella organization for science. Organizations—like the American Association of Pharmaceutical Scientists (AAPS)—are large, industry-type organizations that some students could be involved in very early on in their career. There are also clinical organizations that do clinical research, like the American College of Clinical Pharmacology (ACCP). And then some of the pharmacy organizations have research goals as well. Groups like ACCP, ASHP, and even APhA all have research goals. If you're in those organizations already, you can look for what opportunities they have for students. The other one that's big for supporting research is the American Foundation for Pharmaceutical Education (AFPE). They actually make awards available to students who want to be involved in research called Gateway to Research fellowships, or scholarships, where students can apply. They really want people to be able to test the waters and see if they like research before applying to a PhD program.

There isn't one major organization I think for funding and support, however, the AFPE is a good one to look towards in that regard. When trying to decide on an organization to follow or get involved in as a member, it comes down to your area of interest. I think any pharmacy organization has some research-based goals, but if you find yourself more aligned with the community or hospital or clinical organizations, you could find resource groups within them. If there's a particular faculty member you like working with, or you like what they do, you can talk to them about what organizations they belong to because there are some organizations outside of pharmacy that support research too.

Myself as an example, I'm involved in the American Society for Clinical Pharmacology and Therapeutics (ASCPT), which has a bunch of student opportunities as well. It's a big world when you start thinking about the types of research you could do.

Are there any suggestions you would make to a first-year pharmacy student to better prepare them or give them a good overview, or glimpse, if you will, into the "real world" of being a PhD in pharmacy?

From a research perspective, with the focus of pharmacy specifically, when you have a PharmD, you can do many, many different things, including research. If you choose to do research as a profession, you could go on and get an additional PhD, and that PhD is typically in pharmaceutical sciences, but it also could be in any of the sub areas as well. The biggest thing for young students to do is look for opportunities as early as possible. Right now I have four students who are doing special topics with me that are all starting this process and getting involved in research very, very early on. Those opportunities may be limited experiences, but it's the first step. All the faculty are open to folks exploring very early. Never be afraid to ask because there's a lot of faculty and there's a lot of opportunity around you!

What have you found to be the best strategy for performing "deep work"—that is, focused time spent to efficiently produce quality results to advance your career?

Simply dedicating time for it. Everybody's busy, whether you are in pharmacy school or a faculty member. If you want to meaningfully contribute to something, you have to dedicate the time to it, whether it's an extracurricular activity or you want to go exercise, you have to schedule time for it. If you want to keep up with the reading in a particular therapeutic area or literature, you have to make time for it. If you want to do good research or be a better clinician, you have to schedule time for it. The key thing is to be disciplined and set time aside for the things that you're passionate about.

What overall suggestions would you make to become poised in the profession of pharmacy as a PhD candidate throughout pharmacy school?

As faculty, we try to give research experiences in any way we can and then try to make sure that those research experiences are leading to meaningful outputs. Look for opportunities to contribute, to being involved in things that are bigger than yourself, and meaningfully contribute to them. If you do, then typically your effort will result in things that will help your résumé and your CV, you'll have the opportunity to present your work, maybe do a poster, and maybe even be involved in a paper. When I review an applicant for our PhD program and they already have a manuscript, or presentations, they've worked in a lab through an independent study, or maybe got a job, I know that they know what research is. It makes them a much stronger applicant than someone who thinks they might know but never really tried anything. The key is to definitely get involved.

Do you have any particular story that really solidified that you wanted to continue down the path of research?

Yes! This may sound odd, but when I went to pharmacy school, I intended to be a physician afterwards. I intended to use pharmacy school as a pre-med track and go straight into medical school. Before I did that, I wanted to make sure I was the best pharmacist I could possibly be. It wasn't until I was in my first year of residency when I had a pretty in-depth question about how a disease was working in the pharmacology of the drug and trying to figure out why a patient may have a different response. I then realized that we, as pharmacists, were the best people to answer those questions. The pharmacist knew more than the physician I was talking to when I was looking for answers. I realized it was much more of a team science thing, and pharmacists were better positioned if I really wanted to be a better researcher in pharmacy. The path wasn't to be a physician; the path was to be a scientist—a pharmaceutical scientist.

The other thing that was sort of weird wisdom-wise is my advice to not feel like your path has to be linear. I mean, if I were to spell out all the different training options I went through, it's way longer than you would imagine, but that's not a bad thing. The experiences you collect along the way are all good things. So I did end up earning a pharmacy degree, then went on and did two years of residency. After that, I earned my PhD and then I actually did a little bit of postdoc training afterwards. When I did get my first job, I knew exactly what I wanted to do and I was well-positioned to be able to do it. You can certainly be much more efficient. You do not have to do a residency to earn a PhD, you don't have to do a postdoc, and you don't have to do a PhD if you don't want to do research. But if you want research to be the predominant thing, that is what you do. If research is an interest for you, you need to be able to lead a team to be able to do it well, and it is the best type of training for our breadth and depth of exposure, because you will have four to five years contributing to science. And that skill set is what will make you successful in your future career.

You've obviously been very successful throughout your research career. What are you most proud of?

The team I lead has just created a new pharmacogenomics program at UPMC (University of Pittsburgh Medical Center). We've implemented something that had started in pharmacogenomic testing, measuring someone's DNA to determine if they have variants that impact their drug response. Now it's making its way to the clinic. So, we created one of the first programs in the country that has crossed the finish line in creating a clinical service—a new testing process—and implemented it in the middle of clinical practice. We've been doing it for about two years now. We've tested about sixteen hundred patients as part of the routine care. The provider who is returning those results and making those changes is a pharmacist. So that's a great new role for a pharmacist. And, because of the outcomes that we've collected from that, I think the team can genuinely say that we've made an impact on clinical outcomes. There aren't a lot of times we can say the research we do translates into improving people's lives very directly. This is one of these situations where I really think we are doing it.

Any final thoughts?

Just to reiterate, I think that when most students come in to study pharmacy, they think of the profession too narrowly. Either they worked in a retail pharmacy, and that's where they think pharmacy is, or they worked in one setting and one type of exposure. Pharmacy is a great degree because you can do a lot of things with it. You become a licensed pharmacist and you can do everything from research to working in an insurance company to being an educator to clinical or community practice. There are tons and tons of jobs. Keep your options open. The world of pharmacy is always changing, so the more you learn and the more you experience, the better prepared you can be. No one has a crystal ball of what pharmacy will look like in the future. I think we all agree that it will be different. It'll be less about dispensing and more about caring for patients, so get the experiences that allow you to make those changes and drive the new profession.

How do you feel that pharmacy has changed since you were a student?

I went to a relatively progressive pharmacy school, and it was even clear at the time that there weren't a lot of people who were going to be owning their own pharmacy when they graduated. It also was pretty forward thinking about the roles of clinical skills. I think we learned very early that a pharmacist's role is going to be more than dispensing. I think in terms of how the field has changed, pharmacists have expanded to many more roles. Pharmacists are starting to be reimbursed directly for those skill sets. I think they've become more integral to overall patient care. In the past, it was much more of a narrow role of the pharmacist seen as someone who just worked at the corner drugstore. I'm not that old, but things have changed for sure. I was one of the first PharmD classes from a bachelor's of science degree in my school and there was a vision which has largely been accomplished. There's a lot more clinical care happening now than there was then.

Many thanks to Dr. Philip Empey for his time in sharing his expertise on his roles, responsibilities, and best-practice tips in the specialty niche of pharmacy, and for student pharmacist Shannon Ye, who led this interview.

ACADEMIA

Karen S. Pater, PharmD, BCPS, CDE

Associate Professor, Pharmacy and Therapeutics,
University of Pittsburgh School of Pharmacy

Dr. Pater graduated from the University of Tennessee College of Pharmacy in 1996. Following graduation, she completed an ASHP accredited Primary Care Residency at Shands Jacksonville, formerly University Medical Center, Jacksonville, Florida.

Since that time, Dr. Pater has been caring for patients in the community in a variety of outpatient settings. She is currently an Associate Professor at the University of Pittsburgh School of Pharmacy where she coordinates the Self-Care course, as well as co-coordinating the Introductory Pharmacy Practice Experiences.

In your own words, what exactly is academia as a niche profession in pharmacy?

It's important to note that pharmacy education differs between institutions, however at Pitt Pharmacy, many of the clinical faculty are part of pharmacy and therapeutics and through their clinical practice they are able to bring real-life situations to the classroom for student learning.

What is your role as a pharmacist in academia?

I split my time between my clinical practice and teaching coursework at Pitt Pharmacy. In addition to that, I participate in research.

Why do you enjoy contributing to the profession through this specialty? Tell us what gets you excited about your work!

I really enjoy getting to know the students and being a part of the growth and development of future pharmacists. It is particularly rewarding to see the change in pharmacy students from P1 to P4 year.

What are the current requirements or certifications to practice in the academia niche of pharmacy?

There is no true standard certification in order to teach in a pharmacy school. However, most of the clinical faculty are board certified in their area of practice and translate that expertise into the classroom.

If you could go back to your first day of pharmacy school, and knew that you would end up in academia, what steps would you take to build your professional résumé to best align you for success?

I would recommend finding a mentor in the area of pharmacy that I had an interest in to shadow and learn more about it.

What organizations, publications, or establishments would you recommend to follow to build a strong repertoire and better familiarize yourself with being an effective leader in academia?

It would really help your career path to actively seek opportunities to teach in IPPE and APPE experiences. In addition, seek out opportunities to practice public speaking, whether through course work or experiential learning.

Are there any suggestions you would make to a first-year pharmacy student to better prepare them or give them a good overview, or glimpse, if you will, into the "real world" of pharmacy academia?

One thing often unseen is that clinical faculty often have several commitments with their job outside of teaching courses—it is a multi-layered position.

I strongly suggest as a pharmacy student to seek out mentors and gain several perspectives throughout the process of determining your ideal career.

What have you found to be the best strategy for performing "deep work"—that is, focused time spent to efficiently produce quality results to advance your career?

With focused work, everyone functions differently so it is important to find which strategy best works for you to form effective productivity habits. For me, I work best under pressure, so you could say I am a high-pressure performer.

You have made several phenomenal contributions to the profession—in particular, your Profession of Pharmacy course focusing on over-the-counter counseling with patients through using standardized patients and the QuEST/SCHOLAR-MAC method. How does this method fit into the role of the community pharmacist in providing the best level of patient care while balancing a demanding workload?

The SCHOLAR-MAC technique was initially presented as an APhA CE program and I played a large role in incorporating it into Pitt Pharmacy's course work.

[Editor's Note: As a former student of Dr. Pater's I (Adam) can attest that this was one of the most practical courses in helping me to develop my patient care counseling skills—I still use what she taught me to this day! To learn more about the course structure, check the Resources section at the end of this book.]

What overall suggestions would you make to become poised in academia for the profession of pharmacy throughout a student's time in pharmacy school?

It will best serve you to be open to every opportunity and work to ensure that you get something out of every experience.

Any final thoughts?

If an initial plan does not work out, give yourself permission to change your mind in terms of a career choice—do not become overly frustrated. When it comes to selecting a career path, focus on what you are passionate about and head that way!

Many thanks to Dr. Karen Pater for her time in sharing her expertise on her roles, responsibilities, and best-practice tips in the specialty niche of pharmacy, and for student pharmacist Steven Moretti, who led this interview.

Quickly and accurately assess the patient	**S** ymptoms **C** haracteristics **H** istory **O** nset **L** ocation **A** ggravating factors **R** emitting factors **M** edications **A** llergies **C** oexisting conditions (past medical history)
Establish if the patient is a candidate for self-care once you have identified the medical and drug-related problems	**S** ymptoms **C** haracteristics **H** istory **O** nset **L** ocation **A** ggravating factors **R** emitting factors **M** edications **A** llergies **C** oexisting conditions (past medical history)
Suggest appropriate self-care strategies based on desired therapeutic outcomes (if appropriate)	**S** ymptoms **C** haracteristics **H** istory **O** nset **L** ocation **A** ggravating factors **R** emitting factors **M** edications **A** llergies **C** oexisting conditions (past medical history)
Teach the patient	**S** ymptoms **C** haracteristics **H** istory **O** nset **L** ocation **A** ggravating factors **R** emitting factors **M** edications **A** llergies **C** oexisting conditions (past medical history)

ADMINISTRATION IN ACADEMIA

Patricia D. Kroboth, PhD

Dean, Dr. Gordon J. Vanscoy Professor, Pharmaceutical Sciences,
University of Pittsburgh School of Pharmacy

Dr. Patricia Kroboth is Dean of the University of Pittsburgh School of Pharmacy and the Dr. Gordon J. Vanscoy Professor of Pharmaceutical Sciences. Her experiences in practice, research, teaching, and administration allowed her to transition quickly to the role of dean in 2002. She earned a Bachelor of Science in Pharmacy from the University at Buffalo, and Master of Science and Doctor of Philosophy degrees from the University of Pittsburgh.

She has had an exciting and well-funded research career exploring basic functions and clinical applications of modulation of the GABA receptor and the family of ligand drugs, the benzodiazepines. She was founding director of what became the country's first Clinical Pharmaceutical Scientist PhD Program, a program that continues to prosper at Pitt. After twenty-one years, she closed her laboratory in 2004 and now focuses on her administrative role.

She is Fellow of the American College of Clinical Pharmacy and Fellow of the American Association of Pharmaceutical Scientists. Among her awards is the 2013 American College of Clinical Pharmacology Award for Mentoring in Clinical Pharmacology.

Dean Kroboth has led the Pitt Pharmacy family to a shared vision for the School of Pharmacy, which is now a leader in education, a research school of distinction, and an innovator in the practice of pharmacy, including the pharmacists' role in the community. The school is considered among the elite schools of pharmacy with research that spans from drug discovery to new models of care with the greater goal of improving patient care and outcomes. At Pitt Pharmacy, students and faculty alike are inspired to strive for excellence and set a high bar for achievement.

Prior to becoming Dean, Dr. Kroboth served serially as chair of both departments of the school, beginning with the Department of Pharmacy and Therapeutics in 1988, and then the Department of Pharmaceutical Sciences in 1996.

In your own words, what exactly is pharmacy administration as a niche profession?

Most of us understand that the term administration includes management and/or leadership of people. In many pharmacy-focused cases, the administrative role may be specifically for clinical and pharmacy operations, information management, government affairs, finance, personnel, operations, or executive administration. In pharmacy, further specification is needed because of the many settings where administration can occur, including, but not limited to, chain pharmacy, institutional pharmacy, national or regional organizations, and academia.

What is your role as a pharmacist in administration? Walk us through the meaning and purpose for being a dean.

Deans are the "CEOs" of the schools they lead. In that role, the dean is responsible for all of the elements that fall within the mission of the school. For most schools, the areas of the mission include both professional and graduate education, research and scholarship, patient care, and service within the school, to the broader university, to local communities, and to scientific and professional communities. As an individual who practiced for several years before entering academia, and then developed a scientific career, I have found that my practice and research experiences inform the decisions I make. For me, my meaning and purpose as dean is to create a sense of community among faculty, staff, and students, who together create the environment in which we work. It means making decisions that are guided by moral and ethical principles. My purpose is to foster passion, creativity, and personal growth, and a spirit of teamwork and collaboration in our entire community, and to assure respect for individuals and a culture of genuine inclusiveness.

Why do you enjoy contributing to the profession through this specialty? Tell us what gets you excited about your work!

I enjoy doing what I do because of the ability to make a difference in the lives of people and to develop partnerships that bring about change in the profession and new opportunities in research, and more. Leading a school to continually evolve and innovate is exciting whether the innovations occur in bringing pharmacogenomics to the patients and the classroom, or in teaching. Establishing a culture where the faculty seek to continually evolve the curriculum so that students can personalize their education and develop expertise at a faster rate. Being able to see students and graduates prosper is truly rewarding. A side benefit is that the overall advances that we make results in enhancing the reputation of our programs.

What are the current requirements or certifications to practice in a management role for a pharmacy organization?

The requirements for dean are usually based on previous leadership experiences and the quality of those experiences, plus a terminal professional degree or doctor of philosophy. To be an academic leader, an individual must have demonstrated leadership as well as academic excellence and expertise in a focused area. Outside of academia, often a residency or fellowship exposing someone to organization management is expected. Hospital pharmacy administration also typically has an expectation of residency and/or a master's degree or experience that would identify that person as a leader capable of effectively leading the organization.

If you could go back to your first day of pharmacy school, and knew that you would end up in a management role

in pharmacy, what steps would you take to build your professional résumé to best align you for success?

I would do exactly what I did do—I treated every job as if that was all I ever wanted to do. I loved each and every job I ever had. In each case when I changed my role or location of work, it was only because opportunity knocked. I gave everything I had to every role I have ever had.

What organizations, publications, or establishments would you recommend to follow to build a strong repertoire and better familiarize yourself with being an effective leader for a pharmacy administration?

Excellence in leadership requires certain sets of principles that need to be understood. Some are natural leaders but others can learn. Everyone can learn from seminars, reading books, or practicing de novo to improve leadership skills. Based upon area of administration, different organizations are good. For academic administration, the American Association of Colleges of Pharmacy (AACP) is a place for networking with people in academia and learning principles of academic leadership. Each other area of pharmacy, for example, chain or institutional pharmacy administration, has their own specialized organizations.

Are there any suggestions you would make to a first-year pharmacy student to better prepare them or give them a good overview, or glimpse, if you will, into the "real world" of being an administrator (specifically, dean) of a pharmacy school?

No one should enter pharmacy school wanting or expecting to be dean. You have to develop an interest area in pharmacy that drives you to become an expert. You have to be good at something and then decide that, in addition to that focus, you want to educate the next generation of pharmacists and add to the body of knowledge through your research and scholarship. The key is to have excellence and desire to continually learn in a specific area and then seek out academia.

What have you found to be the best strategy for performing "deep work"—that is, focused time spent to efficiently produce quality results to advance your career?

The academic year starts on time and ends on time, which creates an urgency around teaching and curricular matters. Time to write or do deep work is something that only the individual can make a priority. Two strategies work for me: one is to create a daily habit of deep work in a specific location and at a specific time, which for me is generally at the end of the day. The second was to master the ability to quickly get deep into a project even when only a small pocket of time was available.

What overall suggestions would you make to become poised in a leadership role for the profession of pharmacy throughout a student's time in pharmacy school?

Few people will find their passion or real area of focus while in pharmacy school. That was truly the case for me. While in school, it is important to experience different types of pharmacy, then focus on one area that seems the best personal match and where you have opportunity. Seven years after I graduated from pharmacy school, I went to graduate school to become a director of hospital pharmacy. Once I became a teaching assistant and started doing my master's thesis, I realized that my journey was my reward and that I had found academic pharmacy!

Many thanks to Dr. Patricia Kroboth for her time in sharing her expertise on her roles, responsibilities, and best-practice tips in the specialty niche of pharmacy, and for student pharmacist Daniel Schrum, who led this interview.

ADMINISTRATION IN COMMUNITY PHARMACY

Brian Bobby, PharmD

Vice President of Clinical Services for Rite Aid

Dr. Bobby graduated summa cum laude from the University of Pittsburgh School of Pharmacy in 2003 as a part of an advanced graduation program. He served as class president on the dean's advisory board, held multiple leadership positions within Phi Delta Chi, and was president of the Rho Chi Pharmacy Honor Society.

Dr. Bobby began his sixteen-year career at Rite Aid as a cashier and then as a pharmacy intern. His professional career began as pharmacy manager in Cresson. During his time as a pharmacy manager, he assumed various roles in special projects, such as a pharmacist recruiter for five states in New England, Special Operations Trainer for the Wellness Ambassador Program, and as an Eckerd acquisitions transition project leader. Dr. Bobby was promoted to a pharmacy district manager, where he served for five years, supporting his own district, plus four additional districts in the Pittsburgh market. Dr. Bobby was placed on a leadership fast track and graduated from the Soaring Leaders program at Rite Aid.

In 2013, Dr. Bobby was promoted to Rite Aid Director of Health Alliance, an innovative population health management program. Under his leadership, Health Alliance saw expansion to seven states and demonstrated the ability for community pharmacies to successfully partner with various organizations to improve the triple aim of improving access to healthcare, improving patient outcomes, and lowering the overall healthcare costs.

Dr. Bobby was promoted to his current role as Vice President of Clinical Services, where he is responsible for oversight and management of multiple clinical programs for all 4,500+ Rite Aid Pharmacies. He manages a team of more than forty clinical pharmacists, as well as provides leadership and oversight for the Clinical Drug Information Center in Moon Township.

Dr. Bobby was recognized in 2011 as the Phi Delta Chi Alumni of the Year for the Mu Chapter at Pitt and in 2016 as Phi Delta Chi Mu Chapter Distinguished Alumni of the Year. He also serves as preceptor at the School of Pharmacy, adjunct faculty, and member of the CE Steering Committee and Advisory Board at Bidwell Technical Institute, where he continues to share his passion for clinical services and advancing the profession with future pharmacists.

In your own words, what exactly is pharmacy administration as a niche profession?

I would describe pharmacy administration in community pharmacy as a position that meets the needs of the corporation, individual stores, and employees. In this role, there is less involvement in meeting the needs of individual patients compared to the store as a whole.

What is your role as a pharmacist in administration?

In my role, I address these needs of the individual stores by creating policies, procedures, and training programs that allow the stores to best serve their patients.

Why do you enjoy contributing to the profession through this specialty? Tell us what gets you excited about your work!

I get the most satisfaction from knowing that my strategies for improving patient care at the corporate level will affect a large number patients as opposed to handling individual patient cases.

What are the current requirements or certifications to practice in a management role for a pharmacy organization?

For my practice, I maintain a Pennsylvania and Ohio pharmacy license. In addition, I maintain certifications to not only provide immunizations, but to conduct Rite Aid's immunization training program for pharmacists.

If you could go back to your first day of pharmacy school, and knew that you would end up in a management role in pharmacy, what steps would you take to build your professional résumé to best align you for success?

I recommend pursuing rotations and experiences that allow for a pharmacy student to experience and shadow leadership opportunities in the pharmacy professions. Some chain stores offer corporate rotations that would allow students to gain these types of experiences.

What organizations, publications, or establishments would you recommend to follow to build a strong repertoire and better familiarize yourself with being an effective leader for a pharmacy administration?

I follow publications such as the APhA newsletter, articles from the *Chain Drug Review* and *PharmacyTimes*, along with internal communications at Rite Aid that involve how Rite Aid compares to competitors.

Are there any suggestions you would make to a first-year pharmacy student to better prepare them or give them a good overview, or glimpse, if you will, into the "real world" of pharmacy management?

In addition to valuable rotation experiences, I want to stress the importance of developing effective communication skills at any opportunity. Communication is a skill that is extremely valuable in a management role.

What overall suggestions would you make to become poised in a leadership role for the profession of pharmacy throughout a student's time in pharmacy school?

I would highly advise that students use rotation experiences to take risks in the sense of trying opportunities where they may not feel as comfortable. This will allow students to receive valuable learning that will prove useful later in a career.

Any final thoughts?

As a pharmacy student and future pharmacist, keep your CV current in order to be ready to take advantage of an opportunity. It's essential to really grasp how small of world pharmacy is, so be sure to always build positive professional relations, as you can never predict where paths will cross again in the future. In addition to this, the value of developing good networking skills and actively trying to meet people in the pharmacy field are priceless. I highly suggest that, as a student, you actively seek out good mentors. I feel that this point should have been emphasized to students more back when I was in school, as I came to learn once I graduated, that a good mentor can really have a positive impact on a young career.

Many thanks to Dr. Brian Bobby for his time in sharing his expertise on his roles, responsibilities, and best-practice tips in the specialty niche of pharmacy, and for student pharmacist Steven Moretti, who led this interview.

MANAGED CARE

Brad Stevens, PharmD

Clinical Advisor, CVS Health

Dr. Brad Stevens graduated in 2012 from the University of Pittsburgh School of Pharmacy. While in school, Dr. Stevens was active in the Pitt Academy of Managed Care Pharmacy (AMCP) chapter, serving as chapter vice president during his P3 year.

After graduation, Dr. Stevens completed a managed care residency at CVS Health in Pittsburgh, and also participated in teaching and research activities through the University of Pittsburgh School of Pharmacy.

Currently, Dr. Stevens serves as a clinical advisor in the health plan business unit of CVS Health. He works with health plan clients to help build their pharmacy benefits, from assisting with formulary development to recommending clinical programs to help with financial analysis.

In addition to his primary job functions, Dr. Stevens served as the coordinator in the managed care pharmacy residency at the University of Pittsburgh School of Pharmacy, as well as one of the preceptors for the residency Medicare rotation.

In your own words, what exactly is managed care as a niche profession?

Managed care at a very high level is taking your skills that you learn both clinically and professionally and using them to get care to patients in both a clinically-effective and cost-effective manner. Succinctly put, it is being a steward for the healthcare dollar. It is a weighing of the clinical benefit, but also cost, with a big emphasis on population health. For example, clinical programs are often worked on by managed care pharmacists, such as medication therapy management (MTM) programs. If these clinical programs are used properly, then readmission and healthcare problems are decreased.

What is your role as a pharmacist in managed care?

I serve as a clinical advisor, and in that role, I do not have any direct patient care, but I do interact with many clinicians both internally and externally. Within the role, you can impact the patients on a higher level. This influence presents even through adjudication of claims. Formulary management, as well as criteria and utilization management, are both important activities that I perform in my role. I also help manage MTM programs.

Why do you enjoy contributing to the profession through this specialty? Tell us what gets you excited about your work!

The work changes every single day and you are always learning something new. Every day, you have an idea of what is going to happen, but at the same time, you really do not. Each and every day, a new product could be released or new legislation could be passed. As a managed care pharmacist, you never see the same thing twice. The job is constantly evolving.

What are the current requirements or certifications to practice in a managed care setting as a pharmacist?

Being a licensed graduate from a pharmacy school is most important, but in addition, I recommend a first-year residency to be very helpful. Competitiveness for these programs is at a high level, and is increasing, but a number of opportunities do exist.

If you could go back to your first day of pharmacy school, and knew that you would end up in managed care in pharmacy, what steps would you take to build your professional résumé to best align you for success?

I was lucky enough to find out about managed care within the first week of pharmacy school via AMCP, and so, go to AMCP meetings! They will pair you with mentors within the field and also give guidance for getting residency. I also recommend doing the managed care elective as well as participation in the Pharmacy & Therapeutics (P&T) competition, held annually by the AMCP Foundation. General electives that would be business-geared will also help. As far as rotations, selecting managed care rotations as well as specialty pharmacy settings along with analytics or industry would serve you well.

What organizations, publications, or establishments would you recommend to follow to build a strong repertoire and better familiarize yourself with being an effective pharmacist in a managed care setting?

AMCP membership is highly recommended. They put out a journal fairly often that hits both on managed care and specialty pharmacy. They also send out the *Daily Dose*, which is a daily email from AMCP to keep pharmacists up to date.

Are there any suggestions you would make to a first-year pharmacy student to better prepare them or give them a good overview, or glimpse, if you will, into the "real world" of managed care?

Shadowing and career roundtable events are very important and helpful for establishing a network.

What have you found to be the best strategy for performing "deep work"—that is, focused time spent to efficiently produce quality results to advance your career?

Being organized is extremely important. Keeping a calendar of events and what all is going on in the office and outside are imperative. To be able to lead and be strategic, you must be able to organize yourself, but also be able to share this with others via mentorship. Additionally, documenting everything is extremely important, both on paper and via email.

What overall suggestions would you make to become poised in the managed care niche of the profession of pharmacy throughout a student's time in pharmacy school?

Striving to continually improve both your communication skills and writing skills will both be essential as a managed care pharmacist. Asking questions is also very important as well as being very engaged in the curriculum.

Networking far in advance is also important, especially for creating connections, so start this as early on as possible in pharmacy school!

Any final thoughts?

There are a lot of opportunities in managed care. There are pharmacists who work in a MTM setting and specialty, but then there are also pharmacists in the client development and business side. There are a lot of opportunities if you look for them—it is a very rewarding career path!

Many thanks to Dr. Brad Stevens for his time in sharing his expertise on his roles, responsibilities, and best-practice tips in the specialty niche of pharmacy, and for student pharmacist Daniel Schrum, who led this interview.

PHARMACY LAW

Carl Gainor, JD, PhD

Clinical Assistant Professor, Pharmaceutical Sciences,
University of Pittsburgh School of Pharmacy

Dr. Gainor completed his pre-pharmacy studies at the University of Michigan and then received his Bachelor of Science from the University of Pittsburgh School of Pharmacy. After completing a one-year residency in hospital pharmacy, Dr. Gainor entered the graduate program at the University of Pittsburgh School of Pharmacy, earning Master of Science and Doctor of Philosophy degrees. He then entered the University of Pittsburgh School of Law, graduating with a Juris Doctor degree in 1975. He was admitted to practice in the U.S. Federal Courts in 1975, and in 1979 he was admitted to practice before the United States Supreme Court.

Dr. Gainor maintained a private law practice in Pittsburgh, Pennsylvania, for more than fifteen years, with an emphasis on cases related to health care. He is currently legal counsel to the Pennsylvania Pharmaceutical Association, an assistant professor at the University of Pittsburgh, an adjunct professor at the University of Arizona, and an adjunct professor at West Virginia University. Dr. Gainor has presented more than five hundred lectures throughout the United States on health-related topics including malpractice, risk management, bioethics, and managed care.

In your own words, what exactly is pharmacy law as a niche profession?

I would describe pharmacy law as managing the legal and regulatory aspects of pharmacy in how it relates to patient care and social issues.

What is your role as a specialist in pharmacy law?

In my career, I have worked to translate local, state, and federal laws into effective operations and practices. Drug companies have their own legal departments that work in ensuring compliance in developing, producing, and distributing medications, so this is an opportunity for this niche as well. Currently, I am more involved in the academic side of pharmacy law, providing education to pharmacy students in order get them practice-ready.

Why do you enjoy contributing to the profession through this specialty? Tell us what gets you excited about your work!

While I enjoyed practicing as an attorney, I find teaching students to be very rewarding. One of the roles in my career I enjoyed most was serving as an expert witness in cases involving pharmacy law.

What are the current requirements or certifications to practice as an expert on pharmacy law?

While having attended pharmacy or law school is an expressed requirement of teaching pharmacy law, it is understood that someone in consideration for such a position would have these degrees.

If you could go back to your first day of pharmacy school, and knew that you would end up in law of pharmacy, what steps would you take to build your professional résumé to best align you for success?

Looking back, I was very content on my career progression and so I don't wish that I had made any different career decisions. My experiences as an intern in a retail environment, a PGY1 inpatient residency at the VA, my pursuit of an MS and PhD in economics, and law school, have all served me well throughout my career.

What organizations, publications, or establishments would you recommend to follow to build a strong repertoire and better familiarize yourself with the field of law in pharmacy?

My go-to, most frequent publications are from the American Society for Pharmacy Law.

Are there any suggestions you would make to a first-year pharmacy student to better prepare them or give them a good overview, or glimpse, if you will, into the "real world" of pharmacy law?

First and foremost, you should focus on doing well academically and pursue internships with practicing attorneys. There are some opportunities that allow students to gain state-required intern hours.

Many thanks to Dr. Carl Gainor for his time in sharing his expertise on his roles, responsibilities, and best-practice tips in the specialty niche of pharmacy, and for student pharmacist Steven Moretti, who led this interview.

GERIATRIC PHARMACY

Amy Haver, PharmD, BCPS, BCGP
Director, Inpatient Geriatric Pharmacotherapy Education
UPMC St. Margaret Family Residency Program

Dr. Amy Haver received a Doctor of Pharmacy degree from Duquesne University and a Bachelor of Science degree from Penn State University. She completed a PGY1 pharmacy practice residency at Allegheny General Hospital in Pittsburgh, Pennsylvania, as well as a PGY2 geriatrics specialty residency at UPMC, St. Margaret. She has experiences in transitions of care research and managed care, and belongs to the Allegheny County Pharmacists Association along with local and national geriatrics societies. Dr. Haver participates in daily patient rounds with the Geriatric Inpatient Service and practices at the UPMC St. Margaret Geriatric Care Center.

In your own words, what exactly is geriatric pharmacy as a niche profession?

Geriatric pharmacy involves taking care of older patients and their medication-related needs, as well as being an advocate for safe and effective medication in older adults.

What is your role as a geriatric pharmacist?

I wear a lot of hats in my role, but overall I work with older adults in various levels of care as patients are usually in transition of care. I mainly work on the inpatient service and pay special attention to patients' home medications, inpatient medications, and discharge medications. Working in an outpatient setting as well, and building relationships with patients, is another area of focus in my practice. I routinely work alongside assisted living nurses to make sure the transition of patients' care is smooth to that type of drastic life change. As a pharmacist, I of course ensure that each medication is necessary for the individual. My team provides care at all levels for my patients.

Why do you enjoy contributing to the profession through this specialty? Tell us what gets you excited about your work!

I work with a population that has a lot of medication-related needs and often times they need additional help. Whether it's organizing medication, or coordinating care among providers, I am on a care team that I truly enjoy. I interact with physicians, nurses, social workers, psychiatrists, and various other healthcare professionals. I really love the collaboration and team effort that goes into meeting the individual patient needs. Medications can become so difficult at this age, so transition of care pharmacists are deliberate and good at finding a problem and fixing it for this patient population. Also, I like to make sure that a patient is educated on the medication they are taking. I'm most excited about contributing to the teamwork by bringing my medication knowledge or literature to the table to help solve a medication problem.

What are the current requirements or certifications to practice in the geriatric niche as a pharmacist?

Most people have gotten to this realm of pharmacy from different career paths. In more recent years, the residency-trained pharmacist population is growing; geriatric pharmacy practice as a whole is growing as well. I was the first resident to go through the program in which I currently work, although I do not believe that it is a requirement. For my current position, I believe that a PGY-1 general pharmacy practice residency is recommended, if not required. When you then get into PGY-2 residencies, that is when you will find more specialties. You can further specialize later in your practice to earn Board Certification in Geriatric Pharmacy credentials (BCGP). Additionally, some people gain the experience through Medicare.

If you could go back to your first day of pharmacy school, and knew that you would end up in geriatric pharmacy, what steps would you take to build your professional résumé to best align you for success?

Getting experience in multiple settings is a great step—community, hospital, long-term care, and managed care. All of those experiences deal with various levels of care that impact an older adult. I would recommend getting involved with local organizations and national organizations like the American Society of Consultant Pharmacists (ASCP). If it's available at your pharmacy school, it would benefit you to specialize in a Geriatric Pharmacy area of concentration within the curriculum. Being intentional and thoughtful when choosing your rotations is key to maximize the experience you will gain prior to graduation. With that experience-focused intention, it is optimal for you and the patients by being exposed to older adults through volunteering and helping out throughout your community. This would really help teach you about challenges older adults have and what brings them joy in their free time. Lastly, not being afraid to speak with people currently in positions and find out how they got into this role.

What organizations, publications, or establishments would you recommend to follow to build a strong repertoire and better familiarize yourself with being an effective pharmacist in the geriatric niche?

Local interdisciplinary geriatric societies, such as the American Geriatrics Society and American Society of Consultant Pharmacists, are excellent organizations. It's a great idea to not only be in pharmacist-specific organizations, but also with others directed toward other healthcare professionals. Reading larger publications, like the *Journal of the American Geriatrics Society* (*JAGS*), and other literature that can be applied to older adults, are excellent for staying current in geriatric care. A smaller publication that is also beneficial is the *Annals of Long-Term Care*.

Are there any suggestions you would make to a first-year pharmacy student to better prepare them or give them a good overview, or glimpse, if you will, into the "real world" of geriatric pharmacy?

If you can get into any projects about medication reconciliation or managed care, or work in the community with the older adult population, you should definitely take that opportunity. As you go through school, be sure to think about how you can apply guidelines to older adults. Speak to multiple professionals within the geriatric field, and get as much focused experience as possible.

What have you found to be the best strategy for performing "deep work"—that is, focused time spent to efficiently produce quality results to advance your career?

This is an ongoing process for me honestly, although I have found that the best strategy is trying to be organized, with the biggest leverage of productivity being prioritizing your work. Knowing when you accept interruptions and knowing when you need to set time aside for deep thinking are crucial.

What overall suggestions would you make to become poised in the geriatric niche of the profession of pharmacy throughout a student's time in pharmacy school?

Don't be afraid to talk to people in their day-to-day activities and different roles they serve. Gain varying experiences. Take advantage of what your school has to offer. Stay up to date on current events. Don't only focus on the pharmacy side of geriatric care, but look at medicine through the scope of interdisciplinary care of older adults.

Any final thoughts?

Team-based approaches can best help patients!

Many thanks to Dr. Amy Haver for her time in sharing her expertise on her roles, responsibilities, and best-practice tips in the specialty niche of pharmacy, and for student pharmacist Kathy Monangai, who led this interview.

GERIATRIC PHARMACY AS A COMMUNITY PHARMACIST

Nelson Chan, PharmD, BCGP
Staff Pharmacist at CVS Health

Dr. Nelson Chan PharmD, BCGP, received his Doctor of Pharmacy degree from St. John's University in 2014. He has been practicing for four years as a pharmacist and has more than nine years of experience in community pharmacy. Dr. Chan believes that no matter where you practice pharmacy, the difference you can make is entirely up to you. He believes that you can be just another pharmacist who mindlessly fills prescriptions like a robot, or you can be that pharmacist who truly makes a difference in a patient's life.

In your own words, what exactly is geriatric pharmacy as a niche profession?

Geriatric pharmacy is broad. It can include just about any setting, which was why I decided to get board certified in geriatric pharmacy. As I'm sure you know, it is not necessary to get board certified to work in retail pharmacy, and in a way, it is almost discouraged. I chose to do so because it made me a better pharmacist so I can better serve my patients.

What is your role as a geriatric community pharmacist?

As a community pharmacist, I don't specifically work with the geriatric population alone. However, many of our geriatric patients do have more complicated disease states, and what I've learned from becoming board certified did help me to better evaluate possible drug-drug interactions or potentially inappropriate medications and better answer any questions patients may have about their prescriptions or any over-the-counter medications.

Why do you enjoy contributing to the profession through this specialty? Tell us what gets you excited about your work!

I can't say that I enjoy every single day of my profession, but it can be rewarding when you see patients doing better on a therapy change that you had suggested to their physician, or when patients are grateful that you helped them save money on a prescription by reaching out to a doctor to change a medication. A little effort can go a long way!

Sometimes you can really make a difference with a small change. There have been many cases that possible drug-drug interactions or inappropriate medications were overlooked, especially in geriatric patients, such as a nonselective beta blocker used in an asthma patient. When I bring this interaction up to a patient, they are usually unaware, and often patients notice an improvement in their asthma symptoms when switched to a selective beta blocker.

What are the current requirements or certifications to practice in the geriatric niche as a pharmacist?

In order to get board certified, you need to have practice a minimum of two years with at least half of that time spent in geriatric pharmacy activities.

[Editor's Note: More information about the BCPS process can be found at the Resources section at the end of this book.]

If you could go back to your first day of pharmacy school, and knew that you would end up in geriatric pharmacy, what steps would you take to build your professional résumé to best align you for success?

If I had a choice to start over, I would have chosen to do a residency instead of perusing the path that I chose. It would have kept my options open to working in other settings like hospital or long-term care. Many pharmacists who choose to get board certified in whatever specialty they select do a residency first. It probably took a lot more time for me to study for the BCGP exam because I did not choose this path.

With just about any setting you choose to practice, networking is important. Unfortunately, what matters more is about *who* you know rather than *what* you know. Also, try your best to keep in touch with your preceptors.

What organizations, publications, or establishments would you recommend to follow to build a strong repertoire and better familiarize yourself with being an effective pharmacist in the geriatric niche?

Try to get involved in student organizations, such as ACCP and APhA, as early on in your pharmacy school career as possible.

As I mentioned before, geriatric pharmacy is very broad, so there really is not one specific organization or publication or establishment to follow, but here are a few that may be helpful:

- **Pharmacist's Letter**: easy-to-follow, once-a-month publication that has some really great comparison charts. The monthly publication usually has information about new meds and any important updates of which you should be aware.
- **PharmacyTimes**: excellent monthly magazine in print and online.
- **FreeCE.com**: great online free resource for continuing education options.
- **ASCP webinars on geriatric pharmacy**: monthly updates on their website found at ascp.com/page/webinars
- **ASHP**: resources on geriatric pharmacy.
- **Email subscriptions from organizations of interest**: FDA, Medscape, APhA, and ACCP.

Are there any suggestions you would make to a first-year pharmacy student to better prepare them or give them a good overview, or glimpse, if you will, into the "real world" of geriatric pharmacy?

I would say try your best to get a rotation with a MTM pharmacist, long-term care, or consultant pharmacist. These pharmacists will probably have the most exposure the real world of geriatric pharmacy.

What have you found to be the best strategy for performing "deep work"—that is, focused time spent to efficiently produce quality results to advance your career?

I like to do my work at cafes because I find the least distractions there. I leave my phone, and anything else I would find to be a distraction, in my car and only bring what I need. I generally avoid busy places because it usually gets crowded and noisy.

What overall suggestions would you make to become poised in the geriatric niche of the profession of pharmacy throughout a student's time in pharmacy school?

Try your best to get involved with student organizations. Keep in touch with your preceptors. Be familiarized with guidelines for common disease states like COPD, asthma, diabetes, anxiety/depression, hypertension, heart failure, and anticoagulation.

If your school has an elective for geriatric pharmacy, go for it!

Many thanks to Dr. Neslon Chan for his time in sharing his expertise on his roles, responsibilities, and best-practice tips in the specialty niche of pharmacy, and for student pharmacist Kathy Monangai, who led this interview.

NUCLEAR PHARMACY

Divya Madhu, PharmD
Nuclear Pharmacist at Cardinal Health

Dr. Divya Madhu graduated in May of 2013 from the PharmD program at St. John's University in Jamaica, Queens. She worked in retail pharmacy from 2007, her freshman year in pharmacy school, until 2016, which is when she got hired with Cardinal Health as a nuclear pharmacist.

In your own words, what exactly is nuclear pharmacy, or nuclear medicine, as a niche profession?

Nuclear medicine is for diagnostic purposes, and it involves Single-Photon Emission Computed Tomography (SPECT) imaging. When you do a regular CT scan/MRI, you get just one image that shows you what is happening, but SPECT imaging gives you the anatomy of a specific area of the body and an idea of a process.

The radiation part provides a better way of seeing clearer imaging, as it is mostly for diagnostic methods as a more detailed and precise way to diagnose the patient.

What is your role as a nuclear pharmacist?

I work in a lab where they compound the tools that are injected into patients as far as the imaging portion of the practice is concerned. This includes white blood cell labeling and making iodine capsules for both thyroid treatment and diagnostic purposes.

Why do you enjoy contributing to the profession through this specialty? Tell us what gets you excited about your work!

Working with other professionals in the medical field is a huge benefit. Also, there is a lot of problem solving involved, with a lot of professional information being exchanged. With this comes a huge potential to learn a lot of things every single day! It's really interesting because it is a field of pharmacy that is not really taught in pharmacy school at all! The information comes from people who have been working for long periods of time and are very knowledgeable in the field. Nuclear pharmacy is so different from other parts of pharmacy, so a passion of mine is explaining what I do as a nuclear pharmacist and talking about the profession! Overall, it's very different from what pharmacists are normally known to practice. In working with radiation and generators, it's really about the technique and how professional you can be—there is a lot of skill involved.

What are the current requirements or certifications to practice in the nuclear niche as a pharmacist?

First and foremost, you'll need a PharmD. From there, it depends on the state. Working in New York currently, I have to be an Authorized User (AU). There are two ways of getting this certification: 1. residency— general PGY1 and PGY2 in nuclear medicine then match in a hospital, and 2. hired directly by a company or a hospital looking for someone to fill a nuclear position. They will pay for your education, i.e., an AU course, which can be done online in about three to four weeks. It will require on-site training, necessitating five hundred to a thousand hours; I did half online and half on-site training at Purdue University.

If you could go back to your first day of pharmacy school, and knew that you would end up in nuclear pharmacy, what steps would you take to build your professional résumé to best align you for success?

Without question, it would be to make sure to incorporate a nuclear medicine rotation, as this is probably the most essential part of getting basic background knowledge. To start your career path as early as possible, it all comes down to networking!

That is why, with regards to social media and pharmacy, it is so important to have a LinkedIn profile—if you don't have one, go create it right now! It only takes a few minutes to get signed up, and you can always add content as you go. You can leverage this to reach out to other peers you may not have met yet in person to start the networking ball rolling and keep it going. You can then use this to shadow someone in the field to learn more about their practice and career path.

Along with connecting with other professionals, doing research on your own and finding out what the field is about and what goes on during a regular day all adds up to make a difference in your career success!

What organizations, publications, or establishments would you recommend to follow to build a strong repertoire and better familiarize yourself with being an effective pharmacist in the nuclear niche?

APhA holds nuclear pharmacy-specific workshops and talks held by people on the board or part of the association. Also, I would consider attending ASHP's Midyear Annual Meetings—there is one in the summer and one in the winter. As far as a publication specific to nuclear pharmacy, the *Journal of the Society of Nuclear Medicine* (specific to the United States) is an excellent resource.

Are there any suggestions you would make to a first-year pharmacy student to better prepare them or give them a good overview, or glimpse, if you will, into the "real world" of nuclear pharmacy?

It is not something that is for everyone; a lot of people get intimidated because you are working around radiation. It is a very safe environment! It is not a harmful environment. Being around needles, radiation, and heavy materials, in the clean room, makes practicing aseptic technique very important! You'll need to focus on these things while in the lab.

Doing the same thing every day is one aspect that I actually enjoy about my career! Some people might find some monotony in it, but by building a lot of the same connections, it gives you a boost in terms of progressing within the field.

Try it! Even if it sounds scary or if you are reluctant, just try it!

What have you found to be the best strategy for performing "deep work"—that is, focused time spent to efficiently produce quality results to advance your career?

LinkedIn. Having all of this information available on a professional network makes a much bigger difference than having a CV or résumé. By leveraging social media, it really strengthens skills and qualities without having to sell yourself the way that you would on a résumé or CV. In addition, it's a great way to network—you can find people the same way you would on most social media, including access to recruiters to find other opportunities amidst a saturated field. People tend to be very content and do not leave their jobs in nuclear pharmacy. In order to advance your career, you must know the right people. Reaching out to people, and ensuring that you have a solid CV or résumé, and continually making sure these are always on point, will serve you well long term!
Professors are a great resource—they know people in various fields and can point you in the right direction. With this suggestion, you will want to make good relationships with professors in your first and second year of pharmacy school!

What overall suggestions would you make to become poised in the nuclear niche of the profession of pharmacy throughout a student's time in pharmacy school?

Reach out to the right people. A lot of work as a student is networking—making the right connections and getting a feel for what you want to do when you graduate is essential. Speak to a pharmacist and see if they are—willing to give you a tour. They can show you the lab and what they do—they are willing to help! At the end of the day, it is what you can show that you did to further your career and show that you were interested in the field!

Any final thoughts?

Yes—a lot of people think that when you start pharmacy school, you are going to end up in a community pharmacy, like a CVS or Rite Aid. It is so important to know that there is more to pharmacy school than just that! Do all of the exploring that you could possibly do! It is never too early to start. Your first and second year are the *best* times to explore the different career opportunities. Whatever you can do to stand out from the crowd, this makes a world of a difference! Priorities in pharmacy school for you should include consistently working on your résumé or CV, going big on LinkedIn, and networking on an ongoing basis.

Many thanks to Dr. Divya Madhu for her time in sharing her expertise on her roles, responsibilities, and best-practice tips in the specialty niche of pharmacy, and for student pharmacist Maria Langas, who led this interview.

INFECTIOUS DISEASE

Lisa Keller, PharmD, BCPS

Clinical Pharmacy Specialist, Antimicrobial Stewardship
at WVU Medicine

Dr. Lisa Keller graduated from WVU School of Pharmacy in 2006. She completed a PGY1 Pharmacy Residency in 2007 and PGY2 Infectious Diseases Pharmacy Residency in 2008, both at WVU hospitals. Following residency training, she took an infectious diseases clinical pharmacist position at Yuma Regional Medical Center in Yuma, Arizona. During her time in Yuma, she started an antimicrobial stewardship program and assisted in the development of a pharmacy residency program, which she served as Residency Coordinator and then Residency Program Director. In 2012, she returned to WVU Hospitals and took a position as the Antimicrobial Stewardship Clinical Specialist. She has served as a preceptor, MUE coordinator, and is the current Residency Program Director for the PGY1 Program.

In your own words, what exactly is infectious disease pharmacy as a niche profession?

An infectious disease (ID) pharmacist focuses on the treatment and prevention of diseases of microscopic organisms. Infectious diseases are found in many patients, including general medicine, oncology, and long-term care.

What is your role as a pharmacist focusing on infectious disease?

There are a lot opportunities within the field. You can specialize in ID consult service, antimicrobial stewardship, transition of care, or HIV/HCV, for example. I particularly focus on antimicrobial stewardship.

Why do you enjoy contributing to the profession through this specialty? Tell us what gets you excited about your work!

The education component gets me the most excited about my work, and the collaboration on how infections are treated that improves the care for patients. I also love to serve as a preceptor and teach the importance of correct antibiotic usage and working on projects.

What are the current requirements or certifications to practice as a pharmacist specializing in infectious diseases for a pharmacy institution?

I highly recommend that you pursue both PGY-1 and PGY-2 programs. Certificate programs for antimicrobial stewardships, and newer board certification for ID, are available. In addition, credentialing can occur for HIV patient management.

If you could go back to your first day of pharmacy school, and knew that you would end up as a pharmacist specializing in infectious disease, what steps would you take to build your professional résumé to best align you for success?

Fortunately, microbiology was a prerequisite for my pharmacy school, so that was helpful for my career progression early on. I was also fortunate enough to get involved in different topics with hospital experience. One thing I would have done differently, would be to specialize in more specific projects. If I did, I would have pursued a master's in public health (MPH) at this point.

What organizations, publications, or establishments would you recommend to follow to build a strong repertoire and better familiarize yourself with being an effective infectious disease expert for a pharmacy institution?

ASHP and ACCP are valuable to participate in and collaborate with as an ID pharmacist. ACCP has practice and research networks, also known as PRNS, that can help you meet and learn from other pharmacists. The Society of Infectious Diseases Pharmacists (SIDP) has great resources and programming. The Infectious Diseases Society of America (IDSA) has guidelines and a publication called *Clinical Infectious Diseases*. Infection prevention and epidemiology publications are also useful.

Are there any suggestions you would make to a first-year pharmacy student to better prepare them or give them a good overview, or glimpse, if you will, into the "real world" of an infectious disease pharmacist?

All of the experiences you're given in your first-, second-, and third-year rotations can build upon one another. As a first-year student, ask questions and shadow professionals. Taking advantage of IPPEs and be open-minded to those experiences as you learn will serve you well in strengthening your clinical skills.

What have you found to be the best strategy for performing "deep work"—that is, focused time spent to efficiently produce quality results to advance your career?

When I really want to focus on a project or reviewing literature, I aim to eliminate the distractions. Personally, I do this through listening to classical music.

What overall suggestions would you make to become poised in a role as an infectious disease specialist of pharmacy throughout a student's time in pharmacy school?

ID is found in many patient populations, so learning about different patient populations is important. Take all of those learning experiences you have as a pharmacy student seriously and use them in your practical decisions. For example, in assessing a general medicine patient versus an oncology patient, one will be more immunosuppressed than the other.

Any final thoughts?

ID is a very exciting and challenging field—you're not only looking at drugs, pharmacotherapy, and pathophysiology—you're dealing with another living organism, which makes it challenging. You can learn how to combat many issues with the use of vaccines and general infection prevention techniques.

―――

Many thanks to Dr. Lisa Keller for her time in sharing her expertise on her roles, responsibilities, and best-practice tips in the specialty niche of pharmacy, and for student pharmacist Kathy Monangai, who led this interview.

MEDICATION THERAPY MANAGEMENT

Melissa A. Somma McGivney, PharmD, FCCP, FAPhA

Associate Dean for Community Partnerships, Professor, Pharmacy and Therapeutics, University of Pittsburgh School of Pharmacy

Dr. Melissa Somma McGivney, PharmD, FCCP, FAPhA, is Associate Dean for Community Partnerships and Associate Professor at the University of Pittsburgh School of Pharmacy. Dr. McGivney is committed to advancing pharmacist-provided patient care in the community. She has led the development of numerous innovative patient care, learning, and research initiatives, including the creation of the Community Leadership Innovation & Practice (CLIP) Workshop Series for students, preceptors, and alumni, and the Silver Scripts Program bringing first- and second-year students to Pittsburgh-area senior centers to provide medication reviews under mentorship.

Dr. McGivney initiated the University of Pittsburgh Community Residency, and has served as director for twenty-two community pharmacy residents in partnership with community pharmacy partner organizations. She led the development and coordinates the NACDS Foundation Faculty Scholars Program for community pharmacy faculty nationally, and has been an invited speaker for more than fifty presentations at state and national meetings.

Dr. McGivney has been honored as fellow by both the American College of Clinical Pharmacy and the American Pharmacists Association. She has been recognized by the National Association of Chain Drug Stores as Community Faculty member of the year in 2011, the American Pharmacists Association Community Residency Preceptor of the year in 2012, and the University of Pittsburgh Chancellor's Distinguished Teaching Award in 2015.

Dr. McGivney received her PharmD degree from the University of Pittsburgh and completed an ambulatory care residency at UPMC Presbyterian, University of Pittsburgh. She previously served on the faculty of Wilkes University School of Pharmacy and UPMC St. Margaret Family Medicine Residency Program before joining the faculty at the University of Pittsburgh in 2003.

What is Medication Therapy Management (MTM), in your own words?

Medication Therapy Management (MTM) became a term with the development of Medicare Part D in 2004. The idea was to put a practice through Medicare beneficiaries where pharmacists were required to look at patients with a higher medication burden to make sure that patients could afford the prescribed medications, take them, and that they were safe for the patient.

Over the years, this has become a benefit in Part D, and the term has been focused to Part D patients only.

Today, the official term is Comprehensive Medication Management, which is the same idea that a pharmacist's responsibility includes the entire medication regimen, and assessing for safety and efficacy for patients. Overall, Comprehensive Medication Management equals individual care.

Medication Management Services includes services that get attached in the dispensing process workflow, such as immunizations, point-of-care testing, and medication synchronization. Things are evolving and being added to this service to enhance what the patient is receiving and to streamline the care into one practice. In this way, Medication Management Services equals comprehensive community care.

How can a pharmacy start implementing MTM and how can they start getting reimbursed?

In order to implement MTM within a pharmacy, such that it undergoes a practice transformation, it will require transforming the pharmacist's role to include broader services in the community. A resource and community designed to support this process is the

Community Pharmacy Enhanced Services Network (CPESN), which functions to transform the way pharmacy is practiced in the community setting. It serves as a way to bring together community pharmacists and pharmacies that already provide comprehensive pharmacy services and want to deliver to a broader population and incorporate a payer for reimbursement of provided services.

Currently, CPSEN is composed of twenty-eight state-wide networks in the country, with the Pennsylvania Pharmacists Care Network (PPCN) comprising one of the twenty-eight here in the state where I practice. How this network works is to first assemble the pharmacist and pharmacies, as physical space is becoming important. This is practical both logistically and financially, as the payer isn't willing to pay until they can see that you can manage their population. You need to get pharmacies together first as a priority.

Using my state of Pennsylvania as an example, we assembled 171 community pharmacies in partnership with the Pennsylvania Pharmacists Association (PPA), and as of this interview, 88 of the 171 PPCN pharmacies participating are in contract with Gateway Health, implementing true comprehensive medication management, including pediatric and geriatric populations. Once a contract with a payer is established, they expect enhanced services—not just one visit—and comprehensive care for the patient. For example, if the patient is eligible, the service will include performing a comprehensive medication review, but will offer services *every time* patient comes into pharmacy as an ongoing service. Through carrying out these contracts and services, it not only is beneficial for the pharmacy as a business, but it demonstrates to the community that pharmacy is more than just an entity.

What are the biggest barriers to implementing and how can they be overcome?

The main barriers would include the public perception of what a pharmacist is, provider status, and understanding that patient care is not just by the pharmacist, but by the entire team in a pharmacy.

These can best be overcome by bringing pharmacists together to offer services to the whole population, and supporting pharmacy technicians and other staff in the pharmacy. Everyone in pharmacy should be engaged in patient care, above and beyond getting the product out the door.

A proposed solution to these barriers is the Pharmacy E-Care Plan by the federal government, which is implemented in every dispensing system in the United States. It includes dialogues with electronic health records (EHR) as a tool to begin to change the traditional practice of a pharmacist looking in to an EHR.

In looking ahead for long-term solutions, it is a very important evolution to have IT system do electronic billing, as payers need to accept the bills that come from the E-Care Plan. However, since currently pharmacists do not have provider status, payers do not have the ability to accept from pharmacists, so we must work together in order to overcome this.

Why do you enjoy contributing to the profession through this specialty? Tell us what gets you excited about your work!

I grew up in rural Pennsylvania and saw being in community pharmacy as such an excellent resource for my hometown, as helping people you know is very rewarding. Community pharmacy is a resource for the community, not just in their health, but also well beyond health. In pharmacy school, I saw the opportunity for what we could be doing as pharmacists and asked, *why doesn't every community have this type of pharmacy and services?* That's where this journey for me began in my career!

As a pharmacist, I love learning alongside students and hearing their ideas and thoughts. It's so nice to work with people who are just as passionate about making a difference in the community, and witnessing students get excited about opportunities by seeing what they can do to fix a problem is priceless.

Working with practices who want to do the right thing, but have legitimate barriers, and allowing us to work alongside them to help overcome these, is rewarding to see in practice. Seeing patients receiving great care is the result. There are so many patient stories that are testimonies to this improved care. One in particular as an example was when a patient had been lost to care completely, but then she was reached out to by her pharmacy. They worked with her to get her back on her medications and take care of herself, leading her to a better state of health.

Ongoing research has allowed findings to be shared with the world to further advance this practice of pharmacy and healthcare.

What are the current requirements or certifications to practice in community pharmacy and conduct MTM?

Your PharmD and license, and all that is required by law in your state of practice. It can come down to the designation of your employer and/or payer to have more credentials, as some employers/payers might expect more certifications (i.e., staff training, CE training, certificate from APhA, or internal training from PPCN).

If you could go back to your first day of pharmacy school, and knew that you would end up where you are, what steps would you take to build your professional résumé to best align you for success?

In sharing advice to current students, I recommend that you come to pharmacy school with an open mind! There is such a breadth of opportunities, especially at Pitt Pharmacy, so if someone invites you to experience something, do it with an open mind. The practice of discovery is very important to your college education. We are very fortunate to have such a wide breadth of experiences with a faculty so willing to have students involved in their work, which can serve as enlightening experiences for the students.

What organizations, publications, or establishments would you recommend to follow to build a strong repertoire and better familiarize yourself with the field of community pharmacy?

Pharmacy Today (through APhA) is a magazine with real-life stories highlighted monthly about what pharmacists are doing nationwide, along with legislative and FDA updates. I highly encourage you to get involved in APhA, and locally here with PPA. At least become a member and see what they are pushing out.

The *Journal of the American Pharmacists Association* is also a great resource, and once you have an area of interest, you can follow more specific publications and outlets, but APhA and PPA are great starting places for enriching your career.

Are there any suggestions you would make to a first-year pharmacy student to better prepare them or give them a good overview, or glimpse, if you will, into the "real world" of community pharmacy?

If you have the opportunity to shadow or intern in your area of interest, it is great to have that level of experience. Remember, you can never take back an experience. If it is a great experience, those memories will stick with you forever; if it is a not-so-great experience, you will never forget that either and can learn from it.

It is imperative that you seek to take on leadership roles and get involved with activities. You need to balance what you are learning in school and what is coming down the road via experiential practice. If you do this, it will allow you to experience really good, high-level practices so that they will never say it can't happen. It will also serve to empower you to see that things are possible.

Take advantage of volunteer and leadership opportunities to see what is coming later on down the road in pharmacy.

What overall suggestions would you make to become poised in the profession of community pharmacy throughout pharmacy school?

Get involved in pharmacy through exploring student organizations, ARCOs, electives, and by engaging in shadowing opportunities. Know that everything you do in school sets you up for a career, so ask yourself:

How do I balance time? How do I speak effectively? How do I identify an interest in something?

Developing these life-long skills will set you up for life after graduation! Through getting involved and serving on an ongoing basis, you will learn your own strengths, as well as learn via discussions with others, such as your student peers and professors.

Final thoughts?

Keep an open mind. You will be surrounded by fellow high-achievers, but it is not a competition. We have a culture of teamwork and support in learning, and we can learn a lot from our colleagues, faculty, preceptors, and experiences. Even in your first year of pharmacy school, it is not a competition; it is okay to work to support your colleagues and friends!

Many thanks to Dr. Melissa McGivney for her time in sharing her expertise on her roles, responsibilities, and best-practice tips in the specialty niche of pharmacy, and for student pharmacist Rebecca Wytiaz, who led this interview.

STATE AND NATIONAL ORGANIZATIONS

Patricia A. Epple, CAE
CEO of the Pennsylvania Pharmacists Association

Pat Epple has served as the CEO of the Pennsylvania Pharmacists Association (PPA) since 2002. As the CEO, she oversees the Association's public policy development, strategic direction, government relations advocacy, member professional development, and membership recruitment and retention. Prior to working for PPA, Pat served in similar chief of staff executive roles for both the Pennsylvania Landscape and Nursery Association and the Greater Harrisburg Association of Realtors.

She earned her Certified Association Executive (CAE) designation in 1988, has served as the president of the Pennsylvania Society of Association Executives (PaSAE), was presented with the Society's Award of Excellence in 1997, and has been in association management for more than thirty years. She graduated from Indiana University of Pennsylvania with a degree in Business and Hospitality Management. She has also served in a number of volunteer capacities, including most recently on the Lupus Foundation's Harrisburg Branch Council and the YWCA of Greater Harrisburg. She serves on the Philadelphia College of Pharmacy Board of Visitors, and is honored that the students of the University of Pittsburgh named her an honorary Kappa Psi.

In your own words, what exactly is advocacy? Why is it important for pharmacists to become involved?

Advocacy is legislative or political advocacy in your community and speaking up for changes in pharmacy practice, as well as public awareness of the pharmacist role in their health. The legislative part is important, as nothing will change in pharmacy unless pharmacists band together and advocate for themselves.

Why are pharmacy organizations important? What value do they provide the profession as a whole, and pharmacists as individuals?

Any professional organization exists to protect and advance the profession themselves. There are both state-level and national-stage organizations for this mission. Both are equally important because one cannot do the other's responsibilities. Advocacy is the most important role that organizations play, coming together as one voice for an important cause. Collectively, there is a more of a one-on-one piece where they coalesce and bring pharmacists together on the legislative front, as they will look to the organizations to see what pharmacists think at the individual level—this is where they are heard.

What is your role as a leader for a pharmacy organization?

In my role as the CEO of PPA, I serve through overall administrative aspects, primarily through working with the board of directors to ensure that the staff implements with strategic direction. I also serve as the Chief Lobbyist for the organization. I work on behalf of PPA members at practice centers and pharmacy schools. Also, I oversee follow-through of the PPA staff, actively implementing the proposed and accepted ideas of the organization.

For someone who is new to a leadership role in an organization, or recently got promoted to a position with more responsibility, where do they start? What specific action steps or preparations should they take to solidify a successful term?

When you start a new position, find out as much as you can about the position and topics relevant to the organization. Talk to people within the organization to find out what their thoughts and expectations are of them and the organization in the future. Find where your own strengths and weaknesses align with the future of the organization. It will serve you to efficiently meet members' expectations. An excellent course of action would be to look for mentors and collaborators to build up your network so that you can effectively work with them in the future. We are so heavily reliant on email that we forget the importance of talking to people, so be sure to capitalize on the value of face-to-face interaction when possible. Finding out the best people with whom to collaborate is key in building your professional network.

Why do you enjoy contributing to the profession through this specialty? Tell us what gets you excited about your work!

I am not a pharmacist, so I didn't think I would have a feeling about giving back to the profession, but the excitement I feel is through feeling that I have made a difference in the PPA. I have seen the growth of the organization through the years, and during that time there has always been something different every day. That keeps it exciting. I have worked with three students who have been on rotation with me who now work on the board, so that is extremely rewarding to experience!

What are the current requirements or certifications to lead in a pharmacy organization?

As far as pharmacy organizations go, there is nothing specific in regards to my role. However, there is a national certification known as the Certified Association Executive (CAE) for national organization leaders. It does not only apply to pharmacy organizations, but would certainly benefit leaders in our space. As far as eligibility for a CAE, you can get it after running an association for more than five years. One point to note is that it is not necessary or required that a pharmacist runs a pharmacy organization—me as an example—which can actually be a great asset to the organization. I have found that I bring new perspectives to the conversation focused on pharmacy outside of that scope.

If you could go back to your first day of office as the leader, and knew beforehand that you would end up in that position, what steps would you take to build your professional résumé or experiences to best align you for success?

I have spent my whole career moving toward a key organization leadership role. Over these years I have been professionally grooming myself for this role—not specifically PPA—but as a national organization leader. I prepared myself with association management law, and without a doubt, my steepest learning curve was gaining more knowledge about the profession of pharmacy.

What organizations, publications, or establishments would you recommend to follow to build a strong repertoire and better familiarize yourself with the position of organizational leadership?

There are a ton of resources available for association management. Specifically, I am a member of the American Society of Association Executives (ASAE); Bob Harris has great tools; PPA's program known as LEAD; and the Pennsylvania equivalent of ASAE.

[Editor's Note: I (Adam) was in the LEAD program class of 2017, and if you are in Pennsylvania, I would highly recommend this for both professional and personal development! See the Resources section at the end of this book for more information.]

Are there any suggestions you would make to a first-year pharmacy student to better prepare them or give them a good overview, or glimpse, if you will, into the "real world" of leading a pharmacy organization?

Join organizations and get involved as early as you can! It can be overwhelming and expensive, but it is worth the investment to belong to one national, one state, and one other approach for organizations. It will be so beneficial for your career if you get involved and commit to these organizations seriously. Can you help? Can you lead? Can you be involved? These are things you have to ask yourself. The connections and involvement can help, and seeking out leadership positions within them will help you to narrow down your career options to a specific niche or field of practice. You can also reach out to your faculty of these different organizations as well for guidance and mentorship.

What have you found to be the best strategy for performing "deep work"—that is, focused time spent to efficiently produce quality results to advance your career?

This can certainly be a challenge during the work week, so sometimes deep work has to be done on the weekends. It cannot be work that is just churned out. With emails, staff meetings, and questions, it can be very difficult. There are other times for things like group work. Sometimes I have to shut out different distractions like phone calls and emails to completely focus on work, however I don't like to do that too often. Finding time to balance that and make the time for deep work is absolutely crucial. Above all, you must find time for yourself.

What overall suggestions would you make to a first-year pharmacy student to become poised as an effective leader throughout pharmacy school?

Confidence is crucial. At the same time, do not be *overly* confident. Asking for assistance is needed as well, especially in having different mentors specific to your career goals. Ask for help when it is appropriate. When it comes to specific skills you will need to use as an effective leader, these would involve writing appropriately, speaking appropriately, and presentation proficiency. If those skills are weak, you must look to develop them from resources available to you, such as those on your school campus. The job market in pharmacy will only get more competitive in the next few years, so it is imperative that as a student you find different ways to stand out.

———

Many thanks to Pat Epple for her time in sharing her expertise on her roles, responsibilities, and best-practice tips in a state organization for pharmacy, and for student pharmacist Kathy Monangai, who led this interview.

CREATING YOUR OWN CAREER AS A DREAM BUSINESS

R̲x̲ FILLED: MY DREAM PHARMACY CAREER!

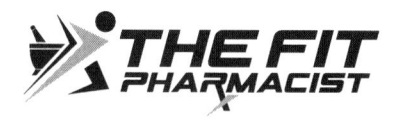

THE FIT PHARMACIST

When I was starting out as a pre-pharmacy student, I was also starting out in the beginning of a physical fitness transformation. As a college student, there was a lot of shiny objects—distractions. Parties, never-ending social outings, and activities unrelated to my goals always seemed to lure my time and attention. I'm going to be honest, in the beginning, that was pretty sweet and a blast! I then came to find through experience that these woohoo diversions of excitement were very short-lived.

As my efforts shifted away from studying and more toward these shiny objects, the academic results were clearly reflected in my not-so-A-student grades. At the same time, the lifestyle of being out late was cutting into my sleeping time and on proper nutrition. By not fueling my body with the adequate nourishment to meet my physical and mental demands, my workouts and health also suffered. The writing was on the wall, as my grades were to the point where my undergraduate academic advisor told me that pharmacy was way too competitive for me, and I should really set my sights toward something more realistic.

That was quite the wake-up call, and it became clear that I needed to take action. It was time to take an honest assessment of what my priorities really were and ensure that my actions were in line with my desired outcomes. This led to profound changes in my life. I put more time into studying, made sleep a priority, and fueled my body with more meaningful nutrition. My grades improved drastically! At the same time, with these same actions, my physical performance during my workouts began to progress, leading to improvements in my physical fitness and physique.

These actions that I committed to as my new lifestyle standard created what I found to be a win-win synergy. Things that benefited my pharmacy career also benefited my physical fitness, and things that fueled my body for peak performance also fueled my brain. This symbiotic relationship for success is what gave me clarity to live my life with both priorities of fitness and pharmacy, and with the magic of compound interest in these endeavors, they led me to personal progress that I had never before experienced in my life.

As I entered pharmacy school, my level of energy, enthusiasm, passion, and performance in and outside of the classroom began to garner attention from some of my fellow classmates. Many were on their own journeys trying to fit in fitness amidst the chaotic pharmacy student life we know all too well (stay in school, you WILL survive).

I was super excited to meet with them and share some simple tips to get them started, as they were able to put these pointers into practice and notice some real results from their effort. Word spread, and soon we were having mini meetings after class. We shared helpful advice with each other on what worked, hashed out some great questions, and formed accountability partners based on common goals and interests.

Right around this time, my good friends founded the Pitt Bodybuilding Club, of which I was super pumped (fitness pun) to join as a founding member. This concept of community, of helping each other and being a source of inspiration and accountability for one another, was so great that is was like a fitness family! I invited my pharmacy friends, and #FitPharmFam began. I went on to become a certified personal trainer through the American College of Sports Medicine (ACSM), and began connecting with others in the profession, who also found irreplaceable value by making physical fitness a priority in their lives.

When I graduated pharmacy school, my focus on becoming even more fit grew, and so I dove deeper with nutrition—not just jumping on some fad diet bandwagon, but really learning evidence-based nutrition on how it can support peak physical performance. Right around this time in 2013, I was getting ready to compete in a drug-free bodybuilding competition, and ended up hiring Joe Klemczewski, PhD, as my prep coach. Joe was one of the most successful lifetime drug-free professional bodybuilders in the world, who also had a renowned reputation of the highest level of integrity in the industry.

I told him about my passion to merge fitness and pharmacy to create sustainable health for not just patients, but for the stress-filled profession of pharmacy, as I witnessed first-hand how much more we can take care of our patients if we first take care of ourselves. His company, The Diet Doc, LLC, which has been successful for more than twenty-five years as of this writing, aims to equip people with the skills to do just that—lead people to better health through science and support with nutrition, mindset, and practical physical activity. Just simplified science that is realistic for the individual's lifestyle, based on a concept he created called *structured flexibility*—having a plan (structure), paired with the ability to pivot through life's variable ups and downs (flexibility).

Joining this company was one of the best decisions I have ever made in my life, as it introduced me to a major concept critical for success that I had neglected up until this point: *mastering your mindset*. What the mind believes, the body can achieve. So, if you want your body to do amazing things, you need to go to the source and get that strong first! Working with Wellness Director and company Vice President Kori Propst, PhD, really opened my mind (pun again) to the true power mindset has on all of the things I was trying to accomplish in my life. I am proud to say that I am still working with both of these amazing mentors today as my business partners and close friends!

Also around this time, social media was growing beyond the

platform of Facebook, and my friends told me you need to get Instagram. As I downloaded the app, it asked me to create an account name. In the moment, I thought of my two biggest passions—fitness and pharmacy—and so created @thefitpharmacist. This was literally where The Fit Pharmacist movement began!

As time went on, people who shared a passion in going above just clocking in as a pharmacist began to connect with me. We all wanted value-focused careers and to improve our own lives through fitness—physical, mental, and nutritional. We also wanted a deeper level of impact and personal power by making fitness a priority. One day, a follower reached out and said he was trying to get his message out and expand his network, so being a lover of writing and networking, paired with a proclivity to puns and alliteration, I got this idea to create what I call a *win-win-win*: write an article highlighting your story and passion sharing what being a Fit Pharmacist means to you, and I would share it on my social media channels on a Friday. We'll call it, #FitPharmacistFriday. What happened next I did not expect.

After that post went live, I got five direct messages (DMs) in less than an hour from both pharmacists and pharmacy students wanting to share their stories. This momentum went on and on, to the point where, as of this writing, I have shared a #FitPharmacistFriday feature every single Friday without fail for more than three years. I don't plan on stopping anytime soon, as we all have a story to tell that will inspire more people than you may realize. If you'd like to be a part of this, please message me on Instagram @thefitpharmacist so I can help to share your message with what is now The Fit Pharmacist community: #FitPharmFam. We'd love to have you and welcome you with open arms!

A Word of Caution—and Motivation!

When it comes to living your life as a Fit Pharmacist, you will meet a lot of naysayers along the way, as I did on my own journey. Many people will tell you that, "You can't do this...the pharmacy is not a healthy environment...you don't have time...." Alone, that *may* seem to hold value until you consider this fact: *what they are saying to you is NOT advice, but merely a reflection of their own limiting beliefs, failures or shortcomings. Ignore the naysayers!*

If you choose not to listen to the limiting beliefs of others, but instead model your outlook after people who *did* make it happen, who live the life you are looking to attain and live yourself, would it not serve you to do the same?

To learn from those who found ways to live their lives to the fullest?

To give their absolute best in their own health and healthcare practice?

Connect with and learn from a group of supportive pharmacists and pharmacy students, who not only inspire others with their own stories of triumph through overcoming personal hardships and obstacles, but even support you along your own journey. *That is what The Fit Pharmacist is all about*—networking, sharing tips and strategies from those who are actually in the trenches walking the talk, and showing evidence that, yes, it can be done!

The Fit Pharmacist is a community within the pharmacy profession to prove you can do it regardless of your work environment, schedule, family situation, or challenges. Not only is there proof, but there's *support* from a community that grows every single day! This may sound like something that would be amazing—a mere fantasy even—and until this community, it simply did not exist in this capacity. That is why it became my life mission to grow it what it has become today:

The Fit Pharmacist is a movement that has extended beyond pharmacy and into all areas of healthcare, so that we can actually care through being healthy ourselves! We guide you to put your health back into healthcare—that is our mission.

That is what healthcare is *supposed* to be! Each needs the help of the other, but the truth is that no one is going to save you, so the best R_x you can fill is yourself through self-care. By taking massive action toward serving others, you will be challenged in all areas of life. Prioritize constant and never-ending improvement on a daily basis. Compound that mechanism of action over time and just imagine what the final yield will dispense to everyone in your life, including you!

There are tons of free resources to get you started on your own journey into fitness, or revv up your current endeavors! Visit www.thefitpharmacist.com and make that your first step to taking control of your life to live it on YOUR terms.

Go forth, be great, and dispense YOUR full potential!

YOUR Dream Career = _____.

(fill in the blank)

Acknowledgments

> *"Each needs the help of the other."*
> —Motto, Phi Delta Chi pharmacy fraternity

This book would not have been possible without the support, guidance, and inspiration from many of my friends and colleagues. I give special thanks to them here:

Patricia Kroboth, PhD, for the conversation we had when I was a P2 that catapulted my passion for innovation in the profession, and for encouraging me to create this resource you are holding in your hands.

Pamela Smithburger, PharmD, MS, BCPS, BCCCP, FCCP, for guidance in structuring this book from the very beginning, and recommendations for key professionals to include in the interview portion of this text.

Kyle McGrath, PharmD, for helping me brainstorm the interview topics and contributing professionals and connecting me with them.

Marcia Borelli, for suggesting some exceptional pharmacy student leaders to be a part of this work in performing the interview process.

Joe Klemczewski, PhD, for his integral work in professionally editing this book and allowing me to gain clarity through simplicity.

To the following pharmacy students who conducted the interviews contained within this book, for their time, dedication, and contribution.

Casey Butrus	**Kathy Monangai**
Maria Langas	**Shannon Ye**
Dan Schrum	**Steven Moretti**
Heather Johnson	
Rebecca Wytiaz	

To the following outstanding leaders in our profession who represented their respective niche in pharmacy and shared their brilliance and insight for pharmacy students of their career path.

Joshua S. Stoneking, PharmD

Heather Johnson, PharmD, BCPS

Gordon J. Vanscoy, PharMD, CACP, MBA

Mike Corvino, PharmD

Richard Waithe, PharmD

Scott R. Drab, PharmD, CDE, BC-ADM

Pamela L. Smithburger, PharmD, MS, BCPS, BCCCP, FCCP

Olufunmilola Abraham, BPharm, PhD

Philip E. Empey, PharmD, PhD

Karen S. Pater, PharmD, BCPS, CDE

Patricia D. Kroboth, PhD

Brian Bobby, PharmD

Brad Stevens, PharmD

Carl Gainor, JD, PhD

Amy Haver, PharmD, BCPS, BCGP

Nelson Chan, PharmD, BCGP

Divya Madhu, PharmD

Lisa Keller, PharmD, BCPS

Melissa A. Somma McGivney, PharmD, FCCP, FAPhA

Pat Epple

Resources

Throughout this book, I have referenced several resources, books, podcasts, articles, and more. To keep these simple, organized, and easy for you to access, I have created a page online listing all of these for you with links to each so that you can access each with one click! Please visit:

www.thefitpharmacist.com/resources

Chapter References

Oath of a Pharmacist
American Pharmacists Association website. https://www.pharmacist.com/oath-pharmacist. Accessed December 23, 2018.

Foreword
Robbins, Anthony. *Awaken the Giant within: How to Take Immediate Control of Your Mental, Emotional, Physical & Financial Destiny*. Simon & Schuster Paperbacks, 2013.

Introduction

(S) Self Mastery

Chapter 1: Clarify Your Why
Pharmacy College Application Service website. http://www.pharmcas.org. Accessed on December 23, 2018.

Pharmacy College Admission Test website. http://www.pharmcas.org. Accessed on December 23 2018.

University of Pittsburgh School of Pharmacy website. http://www.pharmacy.pitt.edu/programs/pharmd/application.php. Accessed on December 23, 2018.

Sinek, Simon. *Start with Why: How Great Leaders Inspire Everyone to Take Action*. Portfolio/Penguin, 2013.

Miller, Donald. *Building a Storybrand: Clarify Your Message so Customers Will Listen*. HarperCollins Leadership, an Imprint of HarperCollins, 2017.

Cardone, Grant. *The 10x Rule: the Only Difference between Success and Failure*. John Wiley & Sons, 2011.

Keller, Gary. *One Thing*. John Murray Publishers Lt, 2014.

Chapter 2: Mold Your Mindset
Robbins, Tony. *Money: Master the Game*. Simon & Schuster, 2016. *Mindfulness: the New Science of Health and Happiness*. Time Books, an Imprint of Time Inc. Books, 2018.

Mark, Gloria, et al. "The Cost of Interrupted Work." *Proceeding of the Twenty-Sixth Annual CHI Conference on Human Factors in Computing Systems - CHI 08*, 2008, doi:10.1145/1357054.1357072.

Dweck, Carol S. *Mindset the New Pscyhology of Success*. Ballantine, 2008. American Psychological Association website. https://www.apa.org. Accessed December 23, 2018.

Gendlin, Eugene T. Ph. D. *Focusing*. Bantam, 2012.

Taren, Adrienne A., et al. "Mindfulness Meditation Training Alters Stress-Related Amygdala Resting State Functional Connectivity: a Randomized Controlled Trial." *Social Cognitive and Affective Neuroscience*, vol. 10, no. 12, 2015, pp. 1758–1768., doi:10.1093/scan/nsv066.

Creswell, J. David, et al. "Brief Mindfulness Meditation Training Alters Psychological and Neuroendocrine Responses to Social Evaluative Stress." *Psychoneuroendocrinology*, vol. 44, 2014, pp. 1–12., doi:10.1016/j.psyneuen.2014.02.007.

Vranich, Belisa. *Breathe: the Simple, Revolutionary 14-Day Program to Improve Your Mental and Physical Health*. Hay House, 2016.

Emmons, Robert A. *Gratitude Works!: a Twenty-One-Day Program for Creating Emotional Prosperity*. Jossey-Bass, 2013.

Puterman, Eli, et al. "The Power of Exercise: Buffering the Effect of Chronic Stress on Telomere Length." *PLoS ONE*, vol. 5, no. 5, 2010, doi:10.1371/journal.pone.0010837.

Naiman, Rubin. "Dreamless: the Silent Epidemic of REM Sleep Loss." *Annals of the New York Academy of Sciences*, vol. 1406, no. 1, 2017, pp. 77–85., doi:10.1111/nyas.13447.

Chapter 3: Self-Care = Healthcare
American Association Colleges of Pharmacy (AACP) Graduating Student Survey: 2017 National Summary Report. AACP Website. https://www.aacp.org/sites/default/files/2017-10/2017_GSS_National%20Summary%20Report.pdf. Published 2017. Accesssed January 19, 2019.

Popkin, Barry M, et al. "Water, Hydration, and Health." *Nutrition Reviews*, vol. 68, no. 8, 2010, pp. 439–458., doi:10.1111/j.1753-4887.2010.00304.x.

Mckiernan, Fiona, et al. "Relationships between Human Thirst, Hunger, Drinking, and Feeding." *Physiology & Behavior*, vol. 94, no. 5, 2008, pp. 700–708., doi:10.1016/j.physbeh.2008.04.007.

Koch, Richard. *The 80/20 Principle: the Secret of Achieving More with Less.* Currency, 2018.

Martin, A. *Rx: YOU! The Pharmacist's Survival Guide to Managing Stress & Fitting in Fitness.* Pittsburgh: CreateSpace, 2018.

Klemczewski J, Propst K. *50 Days to Your Best Life!* Evansville: Word Spank, 2014. Schwartz, David Joseph. *The Magic of Thinking Big.* Vermilion, 2016.

Chapter 4: Tame Time Management with Deep Work

Newport, Cal. *Deep Work.* Piatkus, 2016.

Frisella, Andy. "Win the Day, with Andy Frisella." 30 Oct. 2018, andyfrisella.com/blogs/mfceo-project-podcast/win-the-day-with-andy-frisella-mfceo107.

Zebian, Najwa. *Mind Platter.* Andrews McMeel Pub., 2018.

Chapter 5: Ask for Help PRN

Chanell.baylor. "National Helpline." *Stages of Community Readiness | SAMHSA,* 14 May 2014, www.samhsa.gov/find-help/national-helpline.

Cathy.carr. "Disaster Distress Helpline." *Stages of Community Readiness | SAMHSA,* 22 Jan. 2015, www.samhsa.gov/find-help/disaster-distress-helpline. Suicide Prevention Lifeline website. *Lifeline,* www.suicidepreventionlifeline.org.

"Veterans Crisis Line: Suicide Prevention Hotline, Text & Chat." *Veterans Crisis Line: 1-800-273-8255, Press 1,* www.veteranscrisisline.net/.

"Behavioral Health Treatment Services Locator." *Home - SAMHSA Behavioral Health Treatment Services Locator,* www.findtreatment.samhsa.gov/.

"Buprenorphine Treatment Practitioner Locator." *Stages of Community Readiness | SAMHSA,* www.samhsa.gov/medication-assisted-treatment/physician-program-data/treatment-physician-locator.

Gang.guo. "ESMI Treatment Locator." *Stages of Community Readiness | SAMHSA,* 2 Oct. 2018, www.samhsa.gov/esmi-treatment-locator.

"Opioid Treatment Program Directory." *OTP Directory,* dpt2.samhsa.gov/treatment/.

"Poison Control Center Online Tool and Resource." *PoisonHelp.org,* www.poisonhelp.org/.

Chapter 6: The Value of an Outside Passion

Greenberg, Melanie. *The Stress-Proof Brain: Master Your Emotional Response to Stress Using Mindfulness & Neuroplasticity*. ReadHowYouWant, 2018.

Gawdat, Mo. *SOLVE FOR HAPPY: Engineer Your Path to Joy*. BLUEBIRD, 2019.
Gladwell, Malcolm. *Outliers*. Penguin, 2009.

Chapter 7: Building Your Personal Brand and Your Competitive Edge

Vaynerchuk, Gary. *Crush It!: Why NOW Is the Time to Cash in on Your Passion*. Harper Business, an Imprint of HarperCollins Publishers, 2017.

Newport, Cal. *So Good They Cant Ignore You: Why Skills Trump Passion in the Quest for Work You Love*. Piatkus, 2016.

Vaynerchuk, Gary. *Crushing It!: How Great Entrepreneurs Build Their Business and Influence–and How You Can, Too*. HarperBusiness, an Imprint of HarperCollins Publishers, 2018.

Howes, Lewis. "My Sweaty Pits and a Cat Named Leaf Moose." 2018 10X Growth Conference, 23 Feb. 2018, Las Vegas, Mandalay Bay Convention Center.

(R) Relationship Building

Chapter 8: Master Your Emotional Intelligence

Goleman, Daniel. "What Makes a Leader?" *Contemporary Issues in Leadership*, 2018, pp. 21–35., doi:10.4324/9780429494000-3.

Goleman, Daniel. *Emotional Intelligence*. Bloomsbury Publishing, 2014.
Doran, G. T. (1981). "There's a S.M.A.R.T. Way to Write Management's Goals and Objectives", Management Review, Vol. 70, Issue 11, pp. 35-36.

Fuhrmann, C.N., Hobin, J.A., Clifford, P.S., and Lindstaedt, B. (2013) "Goal-Setting Strategies for Scientific and Career Success." Science Careers. http:// sciencecareers.sciencemag.org/career_magazine/previous_issues/articles/2013_12_03/caredit.a1300263.

Wake Forest University. Office of Personal & Career Development. "SMART Goal Setting Instructions" http://professional.opcd.wfu.edu/files/2012/09/Smart-Goal-Setting.pdf.

Chapter 9: Nurture Your Networking

Cardone, Grant. *Sell or Be Sold: How to Get Your Way in Business and in Life*. Greenleaf Book Group Press, 2016.

Coyle, Daniel. *Culture Code: the Secrets of Highly Successful Groups*. Random House Business, 2019.

"How to Look Confident." *Tonyrobbins.com*, 30 Aug. 2018, www.tonyrobbins.com/mind-meaning/confidence-and-charisma.

Navarro, Joe, and Marvin Karlins. *What Every BODY Is Saying: an Ex-FBI Agents Guide to Speed-Reading People*. Harper Collins, 2015.

Chapter 10: The Three Levels of Mentorship

University of Pittsburgh School of Pharmacy website. http://www.pharmacy.pitt.edu/programs/pharmd/curriculum.php.
Accessed January 23, 2019.

Pharmacy College Application Service PharmD School Directory website. http://www.pharmcas.org/school-directory/#/pharmd/general-information.
Accessed January 23, 2019.

Student National Pharmaceutical Association website. https://snpha.org.
Accessed January 23, 2019.

Ramsey, Dave. *Entreleadership: 20 Years of Practical Business Wisdom from the Trenches*. Howard Books, 2011.

Chapter 11: Leadership & Legacy

Rock, David. "Managing with the Brain in Mind." *Strategy Business*, 27 Aug. 2009, www.strategy-business.com/article/09306?gko=5df7f.

Rock, David. *Quiet Leadership: Help People Think Better – Don't Tell Them What to Do!: Six Steps to Transforming Performance at Work*. Harper, 2007.

Rock, David, and Jeffrey Schwartz. "The Neuroscience of Leadership." *Strategy Business*, 30 May 2006, www.strategy-business.com/article/06207?gko=6da0a.

Cacioppo, John T., and William Patrick. *Loneliness: Human Nature and the Need for Social Connection*. Norton, 2009.

Chapter 12: Build Your Team as a Pharmacy Leader

"SCARF: A Brain-Based Model for Collaborating with and Influencing Others (Vol. 1)." *Neuro Leadership Institute*, neuroleadership.com/portfolio-items/scarf-a-brain-based-model-for-collaborating-with-and-influencing-others/.

Tabibnia, Golnaz, et al. "The Sunny Side of Fairness." *Psychological Science*, vol. 19, no. 4, 2008, pp. 339–347., doi:10.1111/j.1467-9280.2008.02091.x.

Marmot, Michael. *The Status Syndrome: How Social Standing Affects Our Health and Longevity*. Henry Holt, 2005.

Chapter 13: Dispense Your Full Potential as a Leader

Willink, Jocko, and Leif Babin. *Extreme Ownership: How U.S. Navy SEALs Lead and Win*. St. Martin's Press, 2017.

Chapter 14: The Long Game

Ruiz, Miguel, et al. *The Four Agreements*. Center Point Pub., 2008.

About the Author

Dr. Adam Martin earned his Doctorate of Pharmacy degree from the University of Pittsburgh School of Pharmacy in 2012, and has more than eight years of experience working full-time in the community pharmacy setting. He's passionate about empowering other pharmacists and pharmacy students to put the health back into healthcare through leading by example to live their best lives and to inspire others along the way to do the same.

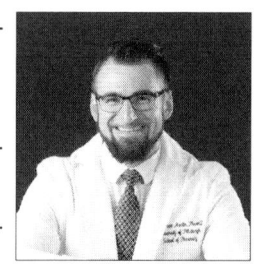

He is the founder of The Fit Pharmacist, LLC, a company with a mission to empower stressed pharmacists with simple, effective plans to master their mindset, nail their nutrition, and fit fitness into their busy schedules. He is the author of the best-selling pharmacy book R_x: *YOU! The Pharmacist's Survival Guide for Managing Stress & Fitting in Fitness* (available on Amazon in print and for Kindle).

As a National Speakers Association (NSA) Professional Speaker, Adam's core passion is traveling to pharmacy schools across the country to speak to pharmacy students, sharing practical plans of action that will empower them to launch their careers and create a competitive edge in the profession to maximize their success and degree of impact.

Through podcasting, collaborating with other passionate professionals, and delivering content across social media platforms such as Instagram, Facebook, LinkedIn, and YouTube, The Fit Pharmacist strives to provide essential tools and resources enabling each and every member of our profession to make a difference in our patients' lives by starting with the source: YOU!

He currently resides in his hometown of Pittsburgh, Pennsylvania, but loves to travel the world with a passion for learning, serving, food touring, and, of course, visiting innovative pharmacy schools and pharmacies along the way.

**Stay connected with me on social media—
I'd love to hear from you!**

Instagram: @thefitpharmacist

Facebook: @FitPharmFam

LinkedIn: linkedin.com/fitpharmfam

YouTube: youtube.com/TheFitPharmacist

Podcast – SoundCloud: soundcloud.com/thefitpharmacist

Podcast – iTunes: The Fit Pharmacist Healthcare Podcast

Twitter: @FitPharmFam